D0077906

# A Color Handbook

# Clinical Endocrinology and Metabolism

### Edited by
## Pauline M Camacho
**MD, FACE**

Associate Professor of Medicine, Division of Endocrinology and Metabolism
Director, Loyola University Osteoporosis and Metabolic Bone Disease Center, Maywood, Illinois, USA

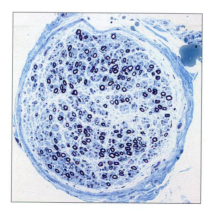

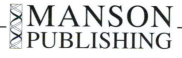
MANSON
PUBLISHING

Dedication:

This book is lovingly dedicated to my family- Francis, Francine, Florence and Paola and to my mother and siblings who all share in my accomplishments.

Copyright © 2011 Manson Publishing Ltd

ISBN: 978-1-84076-121-4

All rights reserved. No part of this publication may be reproduced, stored in a retrieval system or transmitted in any form or by any means without the written permission of the copyright holder or in accordance with the provisions of the Copyright Act 1956 (as amended), or under the terms of any licence permitting limited copying issued by the Copyright Licensing Agency, 33–34 Alfred Place, London WC1E 7DP, UK.

Any person who does any unauthorized act in relation to this publication may be liable to criminal prosecution and civil claims for damages.

A CIP catalogue record for this book is available from the British Library.

For full details of all Manson Publishing titles please write to:
Manson Publishing Ltd, 73 Corringham Road, London NW11 7DL, UK.
Tel: +44(0)20 8905 5150
Fax: +44(0)20 8201 9233
Website: www.mansonpublishing.com

Commissioning editor: Jill Northcott
Project manager: Kate Nardoni
Copy editor: Ruth Maxwell
Proof reader: Susie Bond
Design and layout: Cathy Martin
Colour reproduction: Tenon & Polert Colour Scanning Ltd, Hong Kong
Printed by Finidr, s.r.o., Ceský Tesín, Czech Republic

# Contents

Preface . . . . . . . . . . . . . . . 4
Acknowledgements . . . . . . . 4
Contributors . . . . . . . . . . . 5
Abbreviations . . . . . . . . . . 6

## CHAPTER 1

**Thyroid disorders** . . . . . . . 9
   Jason L. Gaglia
   Jeffrey R. Garber
Normal thyroid . . . . . . . . . . 10
Thyrotoxicosis . . . . . . . . . . . 12
Graves' disease . . . . . . . . . . 15
Hypothyroidism . . . . . . . . .20
Thyroiditis . . . . . . . . . . . . . 22
   Louis G. Portugal
   Alexander J. Langerman
Thyroid cancer . . . . . . . . . . 31

## CHAPTER 2

**Diabetes mellitus** . . . . . . 39
   Amit Dayal
   Mary Ann Emanuele
   Nicholas Emanuele
Introduction . . . . . . . . . . . 40
Retinopathy . . . . . . . . . . . . 41
Nephropathy . . . . . . . . . . . 43
Neuropathy . . . . . . . . . . . . 45
Skin manifestations . . . . . . . 48
The diabetic foot . . . . . . . . 54
Cardiovascular disease
   in diabetes . . . . . . . . . . . 57
Secondary causes of diabetes . 60
Therapeutic options for
   type 2 diabetes . . . . . . . . 64

## CHAPTER 3

**Metabolic bone
disorders** . . . . . . . . . . . . 65
   Cyprian Gardine
   Pauline M. Camacho
Osteoporosis . . . . . . . . . . . 66
Primary hyperparathyroidism  71

Hypoparathyroidism and
   pseudohypoparathyroidism
   . . . . . . . . . . . . . . . . . . .75
Paget's disease . . . . . . . . . . 78
Osteomalacia . . . . . . . . . . . 82
Sclerotic bone disorders . . . . 87

## CHAPTER 4

**Hypothalamic–pituitary
disorders** . . . . . . . . . . . . 91
   S. Sethu K. Reddy
Introduction . . . . . . . . . . . 92
Pituitary adenomas . . . . . . . 92
Prolactinoma . . . . . . . . . . . 96
Acromegaly . . . . . . . . . . . . 99
Cushing disease and ectopic
   ACTH syndrome . . . . . 104
Other pituitary adenomas . . 107
Pituitary apoplexy . . . . . . . 110
Posterior pituitary . . . . . . . 111

## CHAPTER 5

**Adrenal disorders** . . . . 113
   Thottathil Gopan
   Amir Hamrahian
Anatomy and physiology of
   the adrenal gland . . . . . . 114
Adrenal insufficiency . . . . . 115
Primary aldosteronism . . . . 120
Pheochromocytoma . . . . . . 124
Cushing syndrome . . . . . . . 130
Congenital adrenal
   hyperplasia . . . . . . . . . . 136
Adrenocortical carcinoma . . 140
Adrenal incidentaloma . . . . 143

## CHAPTER 6

**Female and male
reproductive disorders** 149
   Rhoda Cobin
   Rebecca Fenichel
Polycystic ovary syndrome . 150
Female infertility . . . . . . . 152

Hyperprolactinemia . . . . . . 154
Secondary amenorrhea . . . . 156
Primary amenorrhea . . . . . 158
Menopause . . . . . . . . . . . . 161
Male infertility . . . . . . . . . 162
Male hypogonadism . . . . . . 163
Gynecomastia . . . . . . . . . . 166

## CHAPTER 7

**Lipid disorders** . . . . . . . 169
   Paraskevi Sapountzi
   Norma Lopez
   Francis Q. Almeda
Lipid disorders . . . . . . . . . 170
Lipoprotein (a) . . . . . . . . . 187
Homocysteine . . . . . . . . . . 187
Future directions . . . . . . . . 187

## CHAPTER 8

**Multiple endocrine
neoplasia,
neuroendocrine tumors,
and other endocrine
disorders** . . . . . . . . . . . 189
   Teck-Kim Khoo
   Mihaela Cosma
   Hossein Gharib
Multiple endocrine
   neoplasia type 1 . . . . . . . 190
Multiple endocrine
   neoplasia type 2 . . . . . . . 196
Carcinoid syndrome . . . . . . 202
Autoimmune polyglandular
   syndromes . . . . . . . . . . 204

**Further reading and
bibliography** . . . . . . . . 206

**Index** . . . . . . . . . . . . . . 213

# Preface

The practice of endocrinology remains an art. Although there have been great advances in biochemical and radiologic testing, the diagnosis of many endocrine diseases still relies on the clinical acumen of physicians. This clinical astuteness is developed after years of seeing many patients with diseases of varying presentations, from mild to severe.

In this book, we aim to transmit knowledge that would otherwise take years of seeing real patients in the clinical setting by providing clinical images from the case files of great clinicians from major teaching institutions. Taking advantage of the internet revolution, some of these images are "borrowed" from websites. We are grateful to the authors of these websites for loaning us their images. The vast majority, however, are images collected from years of experience.

In addition to clinical images, this book also provides helpful tables and algorithms. Contrary to other atlases in publication, this book contains very comprehensive discussions of the diagnosis and treatment pf each of the diseases. Therefore, this colorful, compact and complete book of endocrinology, an essential part of our readers' endocrine libraries.

The authors of this book have worked long and hard on this very important project and it is our wish that through this endeavor, we will improve the science and art of our specialty.

Pauline M. Camacho, MD, FACE
Editor

# Acknowledgments

Chapter 7: The authors wish to acknowledge Kathy Stone and her invaluable technical assistance in preparing some of the images in this chapter.

# Contributors

**Francis Q. Almeda**, MD
Assistant Professor of Medicine
Advanced Heart Group
Ingalls Memorial Hospital, Harvey, Illinois

**Pauline M. Camacho**, MD, FACE
Associate Professor of Medicine
Division of Endocrinology & Metabolism
Director, Loyola University Osteoporosis &
    Metabolic Bone Disease Center
Maywood, Illinois

**Rhoda Cobin**, MD, MACE
Clinical Professor of Medicine
The Mount Sinai School of Medicine, New York

**Mihaela Cosma**, MD
Division of Endocrinology, Nutrition and
    Metabolism
Mayo Clinic College of Medicine
Rochester, Minnesota

**Amit Dayal**, MD
Fellow in Endocrinology
Loyola University Medical Center
Maywood, Illinois

**Mary Ann Emanuele**, MD
Professor of Medicine
Loyola University Medical Center
Maywood, Illinois

**Nicholas Emanuele**, MD
Professor of Medicine and Director,
Division of Endocrinology and Metabolism
Loyola University Medical Center
Maywood, Illinois
& Veterans Affairs Hospital
Hines, Illinois

**Rebecca Fenichel**
Assistant Professor of Clinical Medicine
Division of Endocrinology
New York University School of Medicine,
    New York

**Jason L. Gaglia**, MD
Instructor in Pathology, Department of
    Pathology, Harvard Medical School and
    Physician, Harvard Vanguard Medical
    Associates and Joslin Diabetes Center,
    Boston, Massachusetts

**Jeffrey R. Garber**, MD
Chief of Endocrinology, Harvard Vanguard
    Medical Associates and Associate Professor of
    Medicine, Harvard Medical School, Boston
    Massachusetts

**Cyprian Gardine**, MD
Endocrinologist Private Practice
South Bend Clinic
South Bend, Indiana

**Hossein Gharib**, MD, MACP, MACE
Professor of Medicine, Division of
    Endocrinology, Nutrition and Metabolism
Mayo Clinic College of Medicine,
Rochester, Minnesota

**Thottathil Gopan**, MD
Endocrinologist
Private Practice
Munster, Indiana

**Amir Hamrahian**, MD
Director, Clinical Research
Department of Endocrinology, Diabetes, and
    Metabolism
Cleveland Clinic, Cleveland, Ohio
Assistant Professor of Medicine
Lerner College of Medicine of CWRU

**Teck-Kim Khoo**, MD
Adjunct Assistant Professor of Endocrinology,
    Des Moines University
Adjunct Clinical Assistant Professor of Medicine,
    University of Iowa
Consultant Endocrinologist, Iowa Diabetes and
    Endocrinology Center

**Alexander J. Langerman**, MD
Section of Otolaryngology Head and Neck
    Surgery
University of Chicago Medical Center, Chicago,
    Illinois

**Norma Lopez**, MD
Assistant Professor of Medicine
Division of Endocrinology and Metabolism
Loyola University Medical Center
Maywood, Illinois

**Louis G. Portugal**, MD, FACS
Associate Professor of Surgery
Section of Otolaryngology Head and Neck
    Surgery
University of Chicago Medical Center, Chicago,
    Illinois

**S. Sethu K. Reddy**, MD, MBA, FRCPC,
    FACP, MACE
US Scientific Director, External Medical and
    Scientific Affairs, Merck & Co.
Immediate Past Chairman, Endocrinology,
    Diabetes and Metabolism, Cleveland Clinic,
    Cleveland, Ohio

**Paraskevi Sapountzi**, MD
Endocrinology Associate
Division of Endocrinology and Metabolism
Loyola University Medical Center
Maywood, Illinois

# Abbreviations

| | |
|---|---|
| 5-HIAA | 5-hydroxy-indoleacetic acid |
| 5-HTP | 5-hydroxytryptophan |
| 17-OHP | 17-hydroxyprogesterone |
| ACA | adrenal cortical antibody |
| ACC | adrenocortical carcinoma |
| ACE | angiotensin-converting enzyme |
| ACTH | adrenocorticotrophic hormone |
| ADH | antidiuretic hormone |
| AHO | Albright's hereditary osteodystrophy |
| AI | adrenal insufficiency |
| AIn | adrenal incidentaloma |
| AIDS | acquired immunodeficiency syndrome |
| AN | autonomic neuropathy |
| ANCA | anti-neutrophil cytoplasmic antibody |
| APA | aldosterone-producing adenoma |
| APECED | autoimmune polyendocrinopathy, candidiasis, ectodermal dystrophy |
| APS | autoimmune polyendocrine syndromes |
| ARB | angiotensin receptor blocker |
| ASCVD | atherosclerotic cardiovascular disease |
| BMAH | bilateral macronodular adrenal hyperplasia |
| BMD | bone mineral density |
| β–MSH | β–melanocyte–stimulating hormone |
| CAH | congenital adrenal hyperplasia |
| cAMP | cyclic adenosine monophosphate |
| CBG | corticosteroid-binding globulin |
| CCH | C-cell hyperplasia |
| CEA | carcinoembryonic antigen. |
| CETP | cholesterol ester transfer protein |
| CHD | coronary heart disease |
| CIDP | chronic inflammatory demyelinating process |
| CMV | cytomegalovirus |
| CNS | central nervous system |
| CRH | corticotrophin-releasing hormone |
| CS | Cushing syndrome |
| CSF | cerebrospinal fluid |
| CST | cosyntropin stimulation test |
| CT | computed tomography |
| CVA | cerebrovascular accident |
| CVD | atherosclerotic cerebrovascular disease |
| DDAVP | desmopressin |
| DHEA | dehydroepiandrosterone |
| DHEAS | dehydroepiandrosterone sulfate |
| DI | diabetes insipidus |
| DIT | diiodotyrosine |
| DM | diabetes mellitus |
| DNA | deoxyribonucleic acid |
| DPN | distal sensorimotor polyneuropathy |
| DST | dexamethasone suppression test |
| DXA | dual energy X-ray absorptiometry |
| ERT | estrogen replacement theray |
| FBS | fasting blood sugar |
| FDG | fluorodeoxyglucose |
| FH | familial hyperaldosteronism |
| (F)MTC | (familial) medullary thyroid cancer |
| FNA | fine-needle aspiration |
| FSH | follicle stimulating hormone |
| GAD | glutamic acid decarboxylase |
| GBM | glomerular basement membrane |
| GH | growth hormone |
| GHRH | growth hormone-releasing hormone |
| GIP | gastric inhibitory peptide |
| GnRH | gonadotropin-releasing hormone |
| GRA | glucocorticoid-remediable aldosteronism |
| hCG | human chorionic gonadotropin |
| HDDST | high-dose dexamethasone suppression test |
| HDL | high-density lipoprotein |
| HIV | human immunodeficiency virus |
| HPA | hypothalamic–pituitary–adrenal (axis) |
| HPO | hypothalamic–pituitary–ovarian (axis) |
| HTLV | human T-lymphotrophic virus |
| ICA | islet cell antibodies |

| | | | |
|---|---|---|---|
| IDL | intermediate-density lipoprotein | PRA | plasma renin activity |
| IGF-1/2 | insulin-like growth factor-1/2 | PRF | prolactin releasing factor |
| IGFBP-3 | IGF-1-binding protein-3 | PRL | prolactin |
| IHA | idiopathic hyperaldosteronism | PSA | prostate-specific antigen |
| IL-2 | interleukin-2 | PTC | papillary thyroid cancer |
| ITT | insulin tolerance test | PTH | parathyroid hormone |
| LDDST | low-dose dexamethasone suppression test | PVD | peripheral vascular disease |
| | | RAI | radioactive iodine |
| LDH | lactate dehydrogenase | RAIU | radioactive iodine uptake |
| LDL | low-density lipoprotein | RT | radiation therapy |
| LH | luteinizing hormone | SCS | subclinical Cushing syndrome |
| LHRH | luteinizing hormone-releasing hormone | SERM | selective estrogen receptor modulator |
| Lp(a) | lipoprotein (a) | SHBG | sex hormone-binding globulin |
| MEN | multiple endocrine neoplasia | SIADH | syndrome of inappropriate ADH secretion |
| MI | myocardial infarction | | |
| MIBG $^{123}$ | I-metaiodobenzylguanidine | SMG | submandibular salivary gland |
| MIT | moniodotyrosine | SRB-1 | scavenger receptor B-1 |
| MRI | magnetic resonance imaging | SSRI | selective serotonin reuptake inhibitor |
| mRNA | messenger ribonucleic acid | | |
| MTC | medullary thyroid cancer | TAG | triglyceride |
| NF-1 | neurofibromatosis type 1 | TC | total cholesterol |
| NIH | National Institutes of Health | Tg | thyroglobulin |
| NSAID | nonsteroidal anti-inflammatory drug | TGF | tumor growth factor |
| | | TGF-B | transforming growth factor beta |
| OCP | oral contraceptive pill | TLC | therapeutic lifestyle change |
| PA | primary aldosteronism | TPO | thyroid microsomal peroxidase |
| PAC | plasma aldosterone concentration | TRAP | tartrate resistant acid phosphatase |
| PCOS | polycystic ovary syndrome | TRH | thyrotropin-releasing hormone |
| PET | positron emission tomography | TSH | thyroid-stimulating hormone |
| PHEO | pheochromocytoma | TSHRAb | thyroid stimulating hormone receptor autoantibody |
| PHP | primary hyperparathyroidism | | |
| PKC | protein kinase C | UFC | urinary free cortisol |
| POEMS | polyneuropathy, organomegaly, endocrinopathy, M protein, skin changes | VEGF | vascular endothelial growth factor |
| | | VHL | Von Hippel–Lindau (disease) |
| | | VIP | vasoactive intestinal polypeptide |
| POF | premature ovarian failure | VLDL | very low-density lipoprotein |
| POMC | pro-opiomelanocortin | WHO | World Health Organization |
| PPNAD | primary pigmented nodular adrenocortical disease | | |

# Thyroid disorders

Jason L. Gaglia

Jeffrey R. Garber

**Normal thyroid**

**Thyrotoxicosis**

**Graves' disease**

**Hypothyroidism**

**Thyroiditis**

Louis G. Portugal

Alexander J. Langerman

**Thyroid cancer**

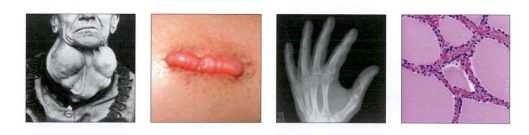

# Normal thyroid

## ANATOMY

During development, the thyroid gland originates as an outpouching of the floor of the pharynx. It grows downward, anterior to the trachea, with the course of its downward migration marked by the thyroglossal duct. The thyroid sits like a saddle over the trachea with the two lateral lobes of the thyroid connected by a thin isthmus, which sits just below the cricoid cartilage. Normally, each lobe is pear shaped, 2.5–4 cm in length, 1.5–2 cm in width, and 1–1.5 cm in thickness; the gland typically weighs 10–20 g in an adult depending upon body size and iodine supply. A pyramidal lobe may extend upward from the isthmus on the surface of the thyroid cartilage and is a remnant of the thyroglossal duct.

The thyroid gland has a rich blood supply with the two superior thyroid arteries arising from the common or external carotid arteries, the two inferior thyroid arteries from the thyrocervical trunk of the subclavian arteries, and a small thyroid ima artery from the brachiocephalic artery at the aortic arch. The venous drainage is via multiple surface veins that coalesce into superior, lateral, and inferior thyroid veins. Blood flow is about 5 mL/g/min but in hyperthyroidism this may increase 100-fold. Other important anatomic considerations include the relative proximity to the parathyroid glands and the recurrent laryngeal nerves.

## HISTOLOGY

The thyroid gland consists of a collection of follicles of varying sizes. These follicles contain a proteinacous material called colloid and are surrounded by a single layer of thyroid epithelium (**1**). These follicle cells synthesize thyroglobulin which is extruded into the lumen of the follicle. The biosynthesis of thyroid hormones occurs at the cell–colloid interface. Here thyroglobulin is hydrolyzed to release thyroid hormones. In addition to the follicular cells are other light appearing cells, often found in clusters between the follicles, called C-cells (**2**). These cells are derived from neural crest via the ultimobranchial body and secrete calcitonin. In adults, the C-cells represent about 1% of the cell population of the thyroid.

## THYROID HORMONE

Thyroid hormone synthesis requires iodide, the glycoprotein thyroglobulin, and the enzyme thyroid microsomal peroxidase (TPO). Synthesis involves several steps including: (1) active transport of I⁻ into the cell via the Na/I symporter; (2) iodide trapping with oxidation of iodide and iodination of tyrosyl residues in thyroglobulin catalyzed by TPO, forming moniodotyrosine (MIT) and diiodotyrosine (DIT); (3) coupling of iodotyrosine molecules to form triiodothyronine (T3) from one MIT and one DIT molecule and thyroxine (T4) from two DIT molecules; (4) proteolysis of thyroglobulin; (5) deiodination of iodotyrosines with conservation of liberated iodide; and (6) intrathyroidal 5′-deiodination of T4 to T3, particularly in situations of iodide deficiency or hormone overproduction.

Thyroid hormones are transported in the serum bound to carrier proteins. It is the much smaller free fraction that is responsible for hormonal activity (typically 0.03% for T4 and 0.3% for T3). The three major thyroid hormone transport proteins are thyroxine-binding globulin, albumin, and transthyretin (thyroxine-binding prealbumin), which carry 70%, 15%, and 10% respectively. A number of conditions and medications can affect carrier protein concentration or binding (*Table 1*). Peripheral deiodinases convert T4 to the more active T3 or inactive reverse T3.

The production of thyroid hormone is normally controlled by the hypothalamic–pituitary–thyroid axis. Thyrotropin-releasing hormone (TRH) produced in the hypothalamus reaches the thyrotrophs in the anterior pituitary via the hypothalamic–hypophysial portal system and stimulates the synthesis and release of thyroid-stimulating hormone (TSH). TSH acts upon the thyroid to increase thyroid hormone production. Negative feedback, primarily via T3 (which may be locally generated from T4 via type 2 iodothyronine deiodinase), inhibits TRH and TSH secretion.

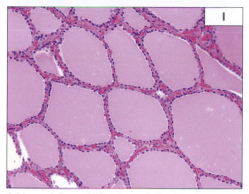

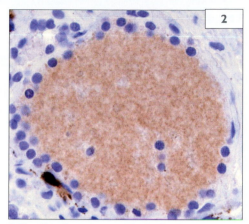

1 Normal thyroid. The thyroid gland consists of a collection of follicles where thyroid hormones are produced and stored. Each follicle consists of central colloid surrounded by one layer of follicular cells. (Courtesy of Dr. James Connolly.)

2 C-cell is demonstrated in the classic parafollicular location with calcitonin staining in brown. (Courtesy of Dr. James Connolly.)

**Table 1  Factors influencing total thyroid hormones levels**

**Increased binding globulin**
- Congenital
- Hyperestrogen states (pregnancy, ERT, SERMs, OCPs)
- Illness: acute hepatitis, hypothyroidism (minor)

**Decreased binding globulin**
- Congenital
- Drugs: androgens, glucocorticoids
- Illness: protein malnutrition, nephrotic syndrome, cirrhosis, hyperthyroidism (minor)

**Drugs affecting binding**
- Phenytoin
- Salicylates
- Mitotane
- Heparin (via increased free fatty acids)

ERT: estrogen replacement therapy; OCP: oral contraceptive pill; SERM: selective estrogen receptor modulator.

# Thyrotoxicosis

## DEFINITION
Thyrotoxicosis occurs when increased levels of thyroid hormone lead to biochemical excess of the hormone at the tissue level. Increased levels of thyroid hormone leading to thyrotoxicosis may result from the overproduction of thyroid hormone (termed 'hyperthyroidism'), leakage of stored hormone from the gland, or exogenous thyroid hormone administration.

## ETIOLOGY
Many cases of thyrotoxicosis are from autoimmune antibody-mediated stimulation (Graves' disease), gland destruction (thyroid-itis), or autonomous nodular disease. Other less frequent causes of thyrotoxicosis include stimulation of the TSH receptor by high human chorionic gonadotropin (hCG) levels, TSH-secreting pituitary adenomas, pituitary-specific thyroid hormone resistance, struma ovarii, functional metastatic thyroid carcinoma, thyrotoxicosis factitia, neonatal Graves' disease, and congenital hyperthyroidism.

Iodine containing drugs such as iodinated contrast agents or iodine rich foods such as kelp may precipitate thyrotoxicosis in susceptible individuals, especially in iodine deficient areas, and is termed Jod–Basedow disease. Amiodarone may precipitate thyrotoxicosis via iodine excess (type 1) or a drug-induced destructive thyroiditis (type 2).

## CLINICAL PRESENTATION
Common symptoms of thyrotoxicosis include palpitations, nervousness, shakiness, insomnia, difficulty concentrating, irritability, emotional lability, increased appetite, heat intolerance, fatigue, weakness, exertional dyspnea, hyperdefecation, decreased menses, and brittle hair. Although weight loss is more typical, approximately 10% of affected individuals gain weight likely due to a mismatch between increased metabolic demand and polyphagia. Due to changes in adrenergic tone, older individuals with thyrotoxicosis may lack many of the overt symptoms seen in younger individuals and instead present with what has been termed 'apathetic thyrotoxicosis'. Often weight loss, fatigue, and irritability are the major complaints in this age group. They may be depressed and have constipation rather than frequent stools. Atrial fibrillation, crescendo angina, and congestive heart failure are also not uncommon in this population.

Signs of thyrotoxicosis include tremors, warm moist skin, tachycardia, flow murmurs, hyperreflexia with rapid relaxation phase, and eye signs. Lid retraction or 'thyroid stare' may be seen with any cause of thyrotoxicosis and is attributed to increased adrenergic tone. True ophthalmopathy is unique to Graves' disease and may include proptosis, conjunctival injection, and periorbital edema. Patients with Graves' disease also typically have a goiter and may have a thyroid bruit from increased intrathyroidal blood flow, while patients with autonomous adenoma(s) frequently have palpable nodule(s).

## DIAGNOSIS/INVESTIGATIONS
Measurement of serum TSH followed by free T4 or T4 index are the initial laboratory studies when thyrotoxicosis is suspected. If free T4 (or T4 index) is normal and TSH is undetectable, a T3 level should be checked to evaluate for T3 thyrotoxicosis. Other laboratory findings that may be associated with thyrotoxicosis include mild leukopenia, normocytic anemia, trans-aminitis, elevated alkaline phosphatase (particularly from bone, but liver alkaline phosphatase may also be elevated), mild hypercalcemia, low albumin, and low cholesterol. A number of medications including dopamine and corti-costeroids may decrease TSH but should not be confused with thyrotoxicosis as the free T4 and/or T3 are not elevated.

Once biochemical thyrotoxicosis is confirmed, the underlying etiology is usually determined by clinical findings or functional and/or structural assessment of the gland. Quantitative assessment of functional status may be obtained with radioactive iodine uptake. An inappropriately high uptake (uptake should normally be suppressed in the setting of a suppressed TSH) confirms hyperthyroidism while a low uptake may be seen with the thyrotoxic phase of thyroiditis, exogenous thyroid hormone ingestion, or thyroid hormone production from an area outside of the neck. A scan with $I^{123}$ or $^{99m}Tc$ pertechnetate can be used to obtain further functional information with images depicting the distribution of trapping within the thyroid gland. Uniform distribution in a hyperthyroid patient most often suggests Graves' disease (**3**). Activity corresponding to a nodule with suppression of the rest of the thyroid suggests a toxic adenoma. A patchy distribution may be seen in toxic multinodular goiter. Structural information may be obtained with physical examination and thyroid ultrasound (**4, 5**). This should be correlated with functional data to ensure that another concurrent process such as thyroid cancer is not overlooked.

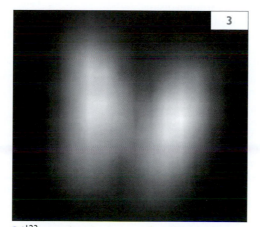

**3** I$^{123}$ scan showing increased and homogenous uptake of radioiodine in Graves' disease.

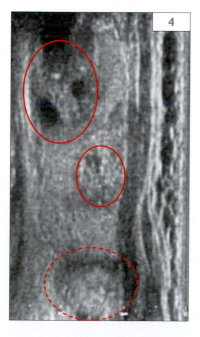

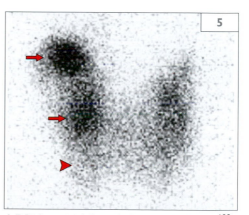

**4, 5** Right sagittal thyroid ultrasound (**4**) and I$^{123}$ scan (**5**) correlation. The superior and middle nodules (circled) on ultrasound correlate with the areas of increased uptake on the scan (arrows) while the inferior nodule (dotted circle) corresponds to a relatively photopenic area and warrants further evaluation (arrowhead). (Courtesy of Dr. Susan Mandel.)

Although the cause of thyrotoxicosis can usually be determined by history, physical examination, and radionuclide studies, in unclear situations the measurement of circulating thyroid autoantibodies may be helpful. A low thyroglobulin level may be useful in differentiating thyrotoxicosis factitia from other etiologies.

**MANAGEMENT/TREATMENT**

Complications of untreated hyperthyroidism may include atrial fibrillation, cardiomyopathy, and osteoporosis. Regardless of etiology of the thyrotoxicosis, beta-blockers, most commonly propranolol, may be used for heart rate control and symptomatic relief. Rate control is particularly important in individuals who have developed an arrhythmia or a rate-related cardiomyopathy. Once a euthyroid state is achieved, the beta-blocker is often stopped. Thyroiditis resulting in thyrotoxicosis is usually self-limiting and often requires no additional therapy, but does carry the potential for subsequent hypothyroidism. In cases of destructive thyroiditis such as amiodarone-induced thyrotoxicosis type 2, steroid therapy may be employed to decrease inflammation. Steroids can also inhibit conversion of T4 to T3.

Thionamides are the major class of drugs used in the treatment of thyrotoxicosis caused by Graves' disease or for usually brief periods in those with multinodular goiter and autonomous adenomas. Commonly utilized forms include propylthiouracil, methimazole, and carbimazole. These agents produce effective intrathyroidal iodine deficiency by inhibiting the oxidation and organic binding of thyroid iodine. Large doses of propylthiouracil may also impair the peripheral conversion of T4 to T3 by type 1 deiodinase. Since these agents inhibit the synthesis but not the release of hormone, they are not useful if there is thyroid hormone leakage from the gland without excess hormone production and also have a latent period before clinical response is seen. Thionamides may cause hypothyroidism, particularly if given in excessive doses over longer periods of time. Potential adverse reactions include rash, arthralgia, myalgia, neuritis, agranulocytosis, hepatitis, and ANCA-positive vasculitis (hepatitis and vasculitis are more common with propylthiouracil), cholestasis (which may also lead to hepatitis is more common with methimazole), thrombocytopenia, and taste disturbance. Rash may occur in as many as 10% of patients, while agranulocytosis occurs in fewer than 1% of patients. This most frequently, but not exclusively, occurs within the first few weeks or months of treatment and is often accompanied by fever and sore throat. Surgery or radioactive iodine may be considered for more definitive therapy depending upon the etiology, clinical situation, and patient preference.

# Subclinical hyperthyroidism

Subclinical hyperthyroidism is characterized by a subnormal serum TSH level and normal free T4 and T3. Subclinical hyperthyroidism is most often asymptomatic and discovered on screening. Several studies report a prevalence of <2% in adult populations. It is generally accepted that once a suppressed TSH with normal free T4 and T3 are detected, this should be reassessed, typically in 2–4 months, to determine if it is persistent or transient and that all patients with subclinical hyperthyroidism should undergo periodic clinical and laboratory assessment. Beyond this, there currently is no consensus as to the management of subclinical hyperthyroidism, but its treatment may be warranted in several sub-populations.

The three major concerns with subclinical hyperthyroidism are: (1) progression to overt hyperthyroidism; (2) cardiac effects, and (3) skeletal effects. In individuals with subclinical hyperthyroidism attributable to nodular disease, there is a high rate of conversion to clinical hyperthyroidism and thus treatment is often considered in this population. In elderly individuals, subclinical hyperthyroidism increases the relative risk of atrial fibrillation threefold, and other adverse cardiac effects including impaired ventricular ejection fraction response to exercise have been reported. Prolonged subclinical hyperthyroidism may be associated with decreased bone mineral density, particularly in postmenopausal women. These risks are considered in developing an individualized treatment plan. In most other individuals, treatment may be unnecessary, and for individuals in which treatment is deferred, thyroid tests are typically performed every 6 months.

# Graves' disease

### DEFINITION/OVERVIEW

Graves', or as it is known in parts of Europe, von Basedow's disease, is an autoimmune disorder in which stimulatory autoantibodies directed against the TSH receptor (TSHRAbs) result in TSH independent stimulation of the thyroid gland causing production and secretion of thyroid hormone. Histologically, hyperplastic columnar epithelium is evident (**6A, B**). Extrathyroidal manifestations may include ophthalmopathy, pretibial myxedema and, rarely, thyroid acropachy. Thyroid enlargement with hormone excess is typical but any of the components, thyroid disease, infiltrative orbitopathy and ophthalmopathy, or infiltrative dermopathy may occur and often run largely independent courses.

### EPIDEMIOLOGY/ETIOLOGY

Graves' disease has an incidence of between 0.3 and 1.5 cases per 1,000 population per year with a female-to-male ratio of between 5 and 10 to 1. The typical age of presentation is between 30 and 60 years. Although it is by far the most common cause of hyperthyroidism in individuals younger than age 40, it is very uncommon in children less than age 10 years. Smoking has been associated with a greater propensity to develop ophthalmopathy and the worsening of ophthalmopathy with antigen release after radioactive iodine therapy.

The thyroid component of Graves' disease is genetically related to autoimmune thyroiditis, particularly Hashimoto's disease, with both often occurring within the same families. The frequency of other autoimmune disorders including type 1 diabetes, pernicious anemia, myasthenia gravis, Addison's disease, Sjögren's syndrome, lupus erythematosus, rheumatoid arthritis, and idiopathic thrombocytopenic purpura is also increased in Graves' disease patients and their families. Although the TSHR is the primary autoantigen of Graves' disease, autoantibodies against TPO and thyroglobulin are also common. Thyroid-directed T-cell-mediated autoimmunity can also be shown. Extrathyroidal TSHR messenger ribonucleic acid (mRNA) and receptor protein have been reported in many other tissues including retro-orbital adipocytes, muscle cells, and fibroblasts and may play a role in the extrathyroidal manifestations not seen in other forms of thyrotoxicosis. Expression may trigger lymphocyte migration into affected tissues. TSHRAbs may be stimulating, blocking, or neutral. Stimulating TSHRAbs bind to the TSH receptor activating adenylate cyclase, inducing thyroid growth, increasing vascularity, and increasing thyroid hormone production and secretion. Changes in the balance between blocking and stimulating antibodies may lead to fluctuations in thyroid hormone levels.

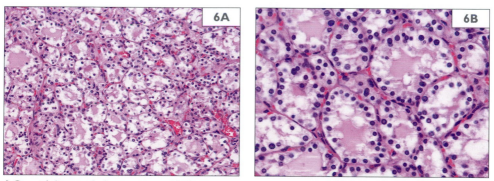

**6** Graves' disease. At lower power (**A**) hyperplastic columnar epithelium with increased infolding is noted. At higher power (**B**) clear vacuoles in the colloid are evident with the increased activity of the epithelium from increased thyroid hormone production leading to scalloping of the colloid. (Courtesy Dr. James Connolly.)

## CLINICAL PRESENTATION

Most patients with Graves' disease have a diffuse goiter. The gland is frequently enlarged two to three times normal but may be much larger. This enlargement is usually symmetric and there is a smooth or lobular surface to the gland. The consistency of the gland may vary from soft to firm and rubbery, but is often more spongy than that seen in Hashimoto's disease. In more 'severe' cases a bruit or thrill may be present with increased intrathyroidal blood flow, which is more common with a larger goiter.

Although thyroid associated ophthalmopathy is closely associated with Graves' hyperthyroidism, either condition may exist without the other; it may predate (20%), coincide with (40%), or follow successful treatment of hyperthyroidism (40%). Thyroid-associated ophthalmopathy results from enlargement of the extraocular muscles and intraorbital fat with an increase in retro-ocular pressure, caused by lymphocytic infiltration, edema, and later fibrosis. This results in proptosis and an impairment of extraocular muscle function. As a result, ophthalmoplegia, diplopia, chemosis, papilledema, or corneal ulceration may occur (**7–11**).

Thyroid-associated dermopathy is seen in 5–10% of patients with Graves' disease and is closely associated with ophthalmopathy. It is generally over the shin (pretibial myxedema), but can be seen over the toes, forehead, neck, or in areas of trauma (**12, 13**). It presents as painless thickening of the skin in hyperpigmented nodules or plaques. Thyroid acropachy,

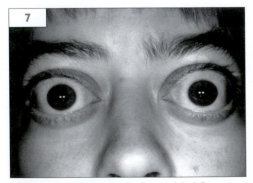

7 Normally, the upper lid is located 1–1.5 mm below the superior limbus, and the lower lid is located at the inferior limbus. This figure demonstrates upper lid retraction (Dalrymple sign) with temporal flare and scleral show in Graves' ophthalmopathy. (Courtesy of Dr. Richard Dallow.)

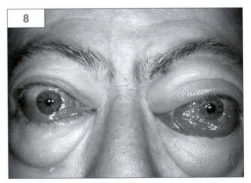

8 Marked periorbital edema and chemosis is demonstrated. (Courtesy of Dr. Richard Dallow.)

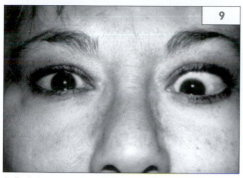

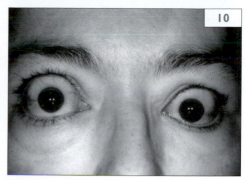

9 Ophthalmoplegia with downward gaze is shown. (Courtesy of Dr. Richard Dallow.)

10 Lid retraction with proptosis and conjunctival injection is shown. (Courtesy of Dr. Richard Dallow.)

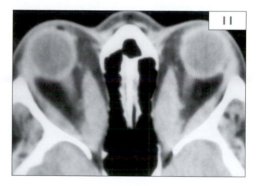

11 Orbital CT demonstrating the classic findings in Graves' ophthalmopathy with thickened recti muscles but sparing of the tendons. Exophthalmos with bilateral anterior displacement of the globes is also shown.

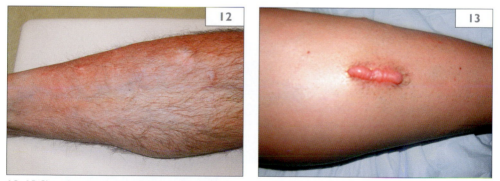

12, 13 Skin changes. Subtle findings of pretibial myxedema with painless thickening of the skin over the shin are shown (12). (Courtesy Dr. Pamela Hartzband.) Thyroid-associated dermopathy is evident as skin thickening after a skin biopsy (13). (Courtesy Dr. Arturo Rolla.)

(clubbing of the digits and periostial bone formation) is seen in less than 1% of patients and is usually associated with longstanding disease (**14–16**). Almost all patients with acropachy also have thyroid-associated ophthalmopathy and dermopathy. Generalized lymphadenopathy, occasionally with splenic and thymic enlargement, may also been seen.

## DIFFERENTIAL DIAGNOSIS

The diffuse goiter of Graves' disease may be confused with the goiter of other thyroid diseases but can often be differentiated based upon laboratory studies or radioactive iodine uptake. Mild bilateral exophthalmos may be familial and also sometimes occurs in patients with Cushing's syndrome, cirrhosis, uremia, chronic obstructive pulmonary disease, or superior vena cava syndrome. Unilateral exophthalmos, even when associated with thyrotoxicosis should raise consideration of another local cause, including orbital neoplasm, carotid–cavernous sinus fistulae, cavernous sinus thrombosis, orbital pseudotumor, or other infiltrative disorders.

## DIAGNOSIS/INVESTIGATIONS

Thyroid tests in Graves' disease are consistent with thyrotoxicosis usually with a suppressed TSH and elevated free T4. Often there is a proportionally greater increase in T3 than T4 concentrations in Graves' disease (this can also be seen with autonomous nodules). If free T4 levels are unexpectedly normal, T3 should be measured to evaluate for T3 thyrotoxicosis.

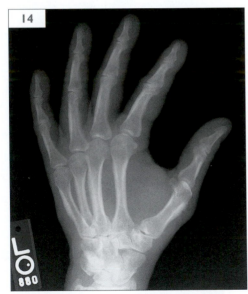

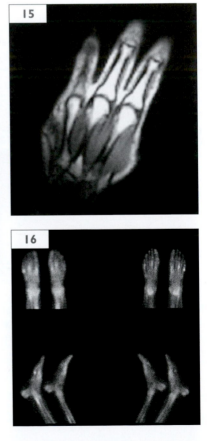

14–16 Thyroid acropachy. Thyroid acropachy is characterized by clubbing of the fingers and toes often with soft tissue swelling over the distal small joints. Soft tissue swelling with periostial or endocortical thickening or subperiosteal reaction may be seen on radiographs (**14**), MRI (**15**), or bone scan (**16**). (Courtesy of Drs. A. Rolla and P. Hartzband.)

Measurement of radioactive iodine uptake may be useful in differentiating Graves' disease, where uptake is inappropriately normal or high, from painless thyroiditis, where uptake is low during the thyrotoxic phase.

Measurement of TSHRAbs is usually not necessary in hyperthyroid patients with Graves' disease with an intact thyroid gland as thyrotoxicosis already serves as an internal bioassay of autoantibody activity. In individuals with possible euthyroid Graves' ophthalmopathy, measurement of TSHRAbs may aid in diagnosis especially if eye findings are unilateral. Similarly, in pregnant women with a prior history of Graves' disease and thyroid ablation, who therefore do not have an internal bioassay of activity, maternal TSHRAbs may be useful in predicting neonatal thyrotoxicosis.

## MANAGEMENT/TREATMENT

The mainstay of pharmacologic therapy for Graves' disease are the thionamides. As described in the thyrotoxicosis section, these drugs inhibit thyroid hormone production. Thionamide drugs may also directly decrease the autoimmunity in Graves' disease by both decreasing antigen expression and cytokine release from the thyroid as well as potential nonspecific immunosuppression leading to decreased lymphocytic infiltration and antigen presentation. Up to 40% of patients previously treated with thionamides remain euthyroid 10 years after discontinuation of antithyroid therapy. Individuals with persistently high levels of TSHRAbs or a T3 to T4 ratio of greater than 20 are more likely to relapse after cessation of antithyroid drugs.

Radioactive iodine is often considered the preferred treatment for patients with Graves' disease in North America and is particularly attractive for those who have relapsed after discontinuation of antithyroid drugs, who would not tolerate a relapse, or are at increased risk of atrial fibrillation due to comorbid conditions or age. Radioactive iodine treatment is contraindicated in pregnant women and those who are breast-feeding. It can induce worsening ophthalmopathy, particularly in smokers, but this risk can be reduced with high-dose glucocorticoid therapy (for example 30–40 mg of prednisone daily, with a taper over weeks to months).

Treatment regimens may vary from center to center and include administering either an ablative dose or a calculated smaller dose of radioiodine. If used, antithyroid drugs are stopped 3–4 days before radioiodine to allow for its effective uptake, and may be resumed 3–4 days after in individuals at high risk for radiation thyroiditis. Since it is radioprotective, pretreatment with proplythiouracil is generally avoided or a higher dose of radioactive iodine is used at time of treatment. Typically, a response is seen within 3 months but since radioiodine may work slowly, it is usual to wait 6 months before giving another dose for persistent hyperthyroidism. By 1 year, permanent hypothyroidism occurs in the vast majority of those given high-dose radioiodine, while those given a lower dose may develop hypothyroidism later and are at higher risk for recurrent hyperthyroidism.

Subtotal thyroidectomy may be preferred in patients with a large goiter, a coexistent thyroid nodule not proven to be benign, or when rapid control is required such as therapy-resistant Graves' disease during pregnancy. Preferably, the patient is treated with antithyroidal agents until euthyroid and appropriate beta-blockade is instituted. Inorganic iodide may be administered for 7–10 days prior to surgery to decrease the vascularity of the gland.

During pregnancy, TSHRAbs, blocking or stimulating, may cross the placenta and affect fetal thyroid function. Regular fetal monitoring for evidence of fetal thyrotoxicosis or goiter is therefore important in cases where the mother has a history of Graves' disease, whether or not there has been prior maternal thyroidectomy or ablation.

# Hypothyroidism

### DEFINITION

Hypothyroidism results from thyroid hormone deficiency in target tissues. Primary hypothyroidism is defined as decreased secretion of thyroid hormone by factors affecting the thyroid gland itself. Central hypothyroidism is due to factors interfering with TSH release from the pituitary (secondary hypothyroidism) or TRH release from the hypothalamus (tertiary hypothyroidism). In rare instances, thyroid hormone resistance may lead to hypothyroidism despite normal or elevated thyroid hormone levels. Hypothyroidism is a graded phenomenon, which in its most severe form can result in myxedema.

### EPIDEMIOLOGY/ETIOLOGY

The most common causes of hypothyroidism are autoimmune thyroid disease, hypothyroidism after surgery, or radioactive iodine. Primary hypothyroidism is relatively common and affects 4–8% of the general population. Hypothyroidism is much more common in women than men with a female-to-male ratio of up to 8–10 to 1. The mean age of diagnosis is mid-50s.

Central hypothyroidism is causal 1 in 20 to 1 in 200 individuals with hypothyroidism, frequently after damage to the hypothalamus or pituitary by tumor, trauma, or an infiltrative disease. Thyroid hormone resistance syndromes are seldom the cause of hypothyroidism with only approximately 1000 registered patients worldwide. Hypothyroidism may also be caused by iodine deficiency (decreased substrate for synthesis) or transiently by iodine excess via the Wolff–Chiakoff effect (inhibition of iodide organification by inorganic iodide excess). Many drugs including lithium, interferon, amiodarone, and antithyroid agents may cause hypothyroidism. Rare causes of hypothyroidism include infiltrative diseases such as sarcoidosis, cystinosis, hemochromatosis, progressive systemic sclerosis, amyloidosis, Riedel's thyroiditis with fibrosis, infectious diseases, thyroid dysgenesis, and consumptive hypothyroidism (excessive type 3 iodothyronine deiodinase activity).

### CLINICAL PRESENTATION

The symptoms of hypothyroidism are often nonspecific and include fatigue, cold intolerance, depression, mild weight gain, weakness, joint aches, constipation, dry skin, hair loss, and menstrual irregularities. Common signs of moderate to severe hypothyroidism include diastolic hypertension, bradycardia, coarse hair, diffuse hair loss (especially the outer third of the eyebrows), dry brittle nails, periorbital swelling, carpal tunnel syndrome, delayed relaxation phase of deep tendon reflexes. Other less common presentations may include yellowing of the skin (carotenoderma), myxedema (pale, waxy, edematous skin without pitting), acropachy, ventricular arrhythmias, and congestive heart failure (particularly in association with underlying cardiac disease). Retarded growth and delayed bone age may be seen in hypothyroid children. In primary hypothyroidism, the thyroid usually has a firm consistency. Its size can be quite variable.

When myxedema coma occurs, it is usually in elderly patients with hypothyroidism and a superimposed precipitating event. Hypothermia, bradycardia, and hypoventilation are common. Ileus is usually present and pericardial, pleural, and peritoneal effusions may be seen. Central nervous system (CNS) manifestations may include confusion, seizures, or coma.

### DIAGNOSIS/INVESTIGATIONS

TSH is elevated in individuals with primary gland failure but may be normal or low in individuals with central hypothyroidism. Although central hypothyroidism is relatively uncommon, free T4 or T4 index should also be checked if this is suspected. Other laboratory findings associated with hypothyroidism may include a normochromic, normocytic anemia or an iron deficiency anemia in the setting of excessive menstrual bleeding, hyponatremia, hypercholesterolemia, and elevated creatine phosphokinase.

## MANAGEMENT/TREATMENT

The standard treatment for hypothyroidism is thyroid hormone replacement, usually with oral levothyroxine (LT4). In primary hypothyroidism, therapy is titrated to a normal TSH (typical goals are 0.3–3.0 µIU/mL) unless otherwise indicated (for example, those with a history of thyroid cancer may have a lower TSH goal). In an adult, full replacement dose is often around 1.6 µg/kg/day. Elderly patients or those with known or suspected cardiac disease are often started on lower doses of LT4 (typically 25 µg/day) and increased slowly until TSH is normal. In central hypothyroidism, trough free T4 or T4 index levels should be followed instead and therapy adjusted as needed to keep troughs in the middle of the normal range. Since the bioavailability of different thyroid hormone brand name preparations are often not equivalent, brand changes should not be made without retitrating the dose. Even if a bioequivalent substitution is made, consider rechecking the TSH in 8 weeks. In general, it takes 6–8 weeks for TSH levels to reach equilibrium after a dose adjustment.

If myxedema coma is diagnosed or suspected, the treatment includes rapid repletion of thyroid hormone deficit, stress doses of glucocorticoids (at least until adrenal function can be evaluated), and treatment of any precipitants. Initially, treatment with intravenous levothyroxine is usually employed as absorption may be variable in the setting of associated gut edema. Intravenous loading dose of 200–500 µg of levothyroxine is commonly recommended, followed by daily intravenous administration of 50–100 µg. Lower daily doses are used in elderly patients and for those in whom myocardial ischemia is likely. The role of intravenous T3 remains controversial and is usually reserved for individuals with low cardiovascular risk with some practitioners advocating additional intravenous T3 at 10 µg every 8 hours for such patients.

Untreated or inadequately treated hypothyroidism during pregnancy may increase maternal and fetal complications including fetal death. Even mild, asymptomatic maternal hypothyroidism may effect cognitive function of the offspring. TSH measurement should be performed before pregnancy or as early as possible during the first trimester for those with known thyroid disease. Since thyroid hormone requirements often increase during the first and second trimesters of pregnancy, in women with known hypothyroidism one strategy has been to increase thyroid hormone dose by about 30% when pregnancy is confirmed and then to follow serum TSH level every 6 weeks during pregnancy to ensure that the requirement for levothyroxine has not changed.

## Subclinical hypothyroidism

Sublinical hypothyroidism is characterized by a mildly increased TSH in the setting of normal free T4 and T3. Subclinical hypothyroidism is most often asymptomatic and discovered on screening. The prevalence has been estimated at between 1 and 10% of the adult population.

The major concerns with subclinical hypothyroidism are: (1) progression to overt hypothyroidism; (2) cardiovascular effects; (3) hyperlipidemia, and (4) neuropsychiatric effects. Individuals with TSH levels >10 µIU/mL or with TSH levels between 5 and 10 µIU/mL and goiter and/or positive antithyroid peroxidase antibodies have the highest rates of progression to overt hypothyroidism and are therefore often treated with levothyroxine. Beyond this, treatment of subclinical hypothyroidism remains controversial.

# Thyroiditis

Thyroiditis rather broadly refers to inflammation of the thyroid gland and comprises a large group of diverse conditions. Since these disorders may be grouped together in various ways and there may be multiple names for the same conditions, these conditions may at first seem confusing. Many of the commonly used names are listed in *Table 2*; the major syndromes are described below and summarized in *Table 3*.

In postpartum thyroiditis, painless thyroiditis, and subacute thyroiditis, inflammatory destruction of the thyroid may lead to transient thyrotoxicosis as preformed thyroid hormone is released from the damaged gland. Due to the destructive nature of these processes, thyrotoxicosis may be preceded by a significant increase in serum thyroglobulin. Reflecting the ratio of stored hormone in the gland, serum T4 concentrations are often elevated proportionally higher than T3 concentrations in contrast to Graves' disease or autonomous adenomas in which T3 may be preferentially elevated. As thyroid hormone stores are depleted and destruction continues, there may be progression to overt hypothyroidism. Hashimoto's thyroiditis, painless thyroiditis, and postpartum thyroiditis all have an autoimmune basis.

## Hashimoto's thyroiditis

Hashimoto's thyroiditis often begins clinically with gradual enlargement of the thyroid gland and eventual development of hypothyroidism. If untreated, the goiter may slowly increase in size. The goiter is diffuse and firm with the gland variably being normal to four times normal size at diagnosis. Associated pain and tenderness are unusual but may be present. In addition to the symptoms of hypothyroidism, about one-quarter of patients with Hashimoto's thyroidits develop other musculoskeletal complaints including chest pain, fibrositis, or arthritis.

Antithyroid autoantibodies are detectable in more than 95% of patients with Hashimoto's thyroiditis with high serum TPO antibodies present in 90% of patients and high serum thyroglobulin antibodies detectable in 50–80% of patients. Elevated antibodies may also be detected in 5–15% of the general population, the majority of whom have normal thyroid function. The ultrasound appearance of the gland is remarkable for a heterogenous echotexture often with multiple ill-defined hypoechoic patches or pseudonodules. Histology often reveals lymphocytic infiltration with germinal center formation and fibrosis (**17**). Radioactive iodine (RAI) scan contributes little to the diagnosis. Uptake may be low, normal, or elevated with an irregular pattern.

With the institution of LT4 treatment, goiter size often decreases within months, whether the patient is euthyroid or hypothyroid. This is especially true in younger individuals as there is likely less fibrosis present. If the goiter is small and the patient is euthyroid and asymptomatic

| Table 2 Forms of thyroiditis | |
|---|---|
| **Type** | **Other names or subtypes** |
| Hashimoto's thyroiditis | Chronic lymphocytic thyroiditis<br>Chronic autoimmune thyroiditis<br>Lymphadenoid goiter<br>Struma lymphomatosa |
| Postpartum thyroiditis | Painless postpartum thyroidits<br>Subacute lymphocytic thyroiditis |
| Silent thyroiditis | Painless (sporadic) thyroiditis<br>Subacute lymphocytic thyroiditis |
| Subacute thyroiditis | Painful subacute thyroiditis<br>De Quervain's thyroiditis<br>(Subacute) granulomatous thyroiditis<br>Giant-cell thyroiditis |
| Suppurative thyroiditis | Infectious thyroiditis<br>Pyogenic thyroiditis<br>Bacterial thyroiditis<br>Acute (suppurative) thyroiditis |
| Riedel's thyroiditis | Reidel's struma<br>Fibrous thyroiditis |
| Drug-induced | Amiodarone<br>Lithium<br>Interferon-alpha<br>Interleukin 2<br>Sunitinib |
| Other | Radiation-induced<br>Traumatic |

no treatment is required. Although controversial, some physicians consider therapy if the TSH is elevated and free T4 is normal since the eventual onset of hypothyroidism is likely in such patients (estimated at 2–5% per year). Antibody levels may spontaneously dissipate and up to 20% of initially hypothyroid patients will later recover and have normal thyroid function if thyroid hormone withdrawal is attempted.

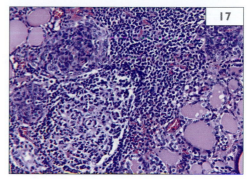

**17** Hashimoto's thyroiditis. There is a profuse mononuclear infiltrate with germinal center formation. Thyroid follicles are small and reduced in number. (Courtesy of Dr. Tad Wieczorek.)

**Table 3 Overview of thyroiditis syndromes**

| Characteristic | Hashimoto's thyroiditis | Postpartum thyroiditis | Silent thyroiditis | Subacute thyroiditis | Suppurative thyroiditis | Riedel's thyroiditis |
|---|---|---|---|---|---|---|
| Thyroid pain | No | No | No | Yes | Yes | No |
| Typical neck exam | Firm symmetric goiter | Small, nontender gland | Small, nontender gland | Tender and swollen gland | Tender thyroid mass | Rock-hard, fixed, painless gland |
| Sex ratio (F:M) | 8–15:1 | -- | 2:1 | 5:1 | 1:1 | 3–4:1 |
| Cause | Autoimmune | Autoimmune | Autoimmune | ? Viral | Infectious | Unknown |
| Associations | HLA DR3, DR4, DR5 | HLA DR3, DR5 | HLA DR3 | HLA Bw-35 | Pre-existing thyroid disease immuno-compromised; structural abnormalities | Systemic fibrosis; hypopara-thyroidism from fibrosis |
| Temporal course | Chronic | Episodic: 70% recurrence with pregnancy | Episodic: recurrence rate unknown | Episodic: <2–4% recurrence rate | May be fatal if untreated | Progressive |
| ESR | Normal | Normal | Normal | Elevated | Elevated | Normal |
| TPO antibodies | Elevated | Elevated | Elevated | Transient mild increase | Absent | Elevated in 2/3 of patients |
| Thyroid hormonal status | Hypothyroid or euthyroid | Thyrotoxic, hypothyroid, or both | Thyrotoxic, hypothyroid, or both | Thyrotoxic, hypothyroid, or both | Usually euthyroid | Euthyroid but may progress to hypothyroid |
| Histology | Lymphocytic infiltrate, germinal centers, fibrosis | Lymphocytic infiltrate | Lymphocytic infiltrate | Giant cells, granulomas | Abscess | Dense fibrosis |
| Typical treatments | Levothyroxine or observation | Observation/variable | Observation/variable | NSAIDs or glucocorticoids | Surgical abscess drainage and antibiotics | Surgery, glucocorti-coids, tamoxifen, methotrexate |

NSAID: nonsteroidal anti-inflammatory drug.

## Postpartum and painless thyroiditis

Postpartum thyroiditis is most common in women with a high serum TPO antibody concentration in the first trimester of pregnancy or immediately after delivery. Women with type 1 diabetes are at particular risk with up to 25% developing postpartum thyroiditis. Thyotoxicosis typically is noted by 3–4 months after delivery and lasts 1–2 months. This may be followed by a hypothyroid phase lasting 4–6 months. There is recovery of normal thyroid function within a year in 80% of women; however, 50% of affected women develop chronic hypothyroidism within 7 years. There is about a 70% chance of recurrence with subsequent pregnancies.

Other than the lack of a temporal relationship with pregnancy, the presentation and clinical course of painless thyroiditis is similar to that of postpartum thyroiditis. About 50% of individuals with painless thyroiditis will have a small, firm, nontender gland and about 20% of affected individuals will develop chronic hypothyroidism. An elevated serum TPO antibody titer is detectable in about 50% of individuals with painless thyroiditis at time of presentation. The titers are on average lower than those seen in Hashimoto's thyroiditis but cannot be used to distinguish the two on an individual basis. A low or undetectable RAIU can usually differentiate thyroiditis from other forms of thyrotoxicosis with suppressed TSH; however, during the recovery phase of thyroiditis, RAIU may be normal or elevated and can be potentially misleading if not correlated with TSH and thyroid hormone levels. On ultrasound, the gland is usually hypoechogenic with normal-to-low vascularity. Histology is remarkable for a lymphocytic infiltrate.

If thyrotoxicosis is present, beta-blockers may be used for symptomatic relief. Since there is not an actual increase in thyroid hormone production, but instead release of thyroid hormone with damage to the gland, thionamides should not be used. If chronic hypothyroidism develops LT4 therapy may be required. Transient hypothyroidism usually does not require additional therapy.

## Painful subacute thyroiditis

Subacute thyroiditis frequently follows an upper respiratory tract infection or sore throat and begins with a prodrome of generalized myalgia, pharyngitis, low-grade fever, and fatigue. With the development of fever, severe neck pain often with swelling is noted. Approximately half of affected individuals develop symptomatic thyrotoxicosis which may last several weeks, and hypothyroidism may subsequently develop. Five percent of patients develop chronic hypothyroidism, usually mild, while the rest have normalization over 6–12 months. The recurrence rate is estimated to be between 2 and 4%. On histology and cytology, giant cells and granulomas may be seen (**18A, B**).

The treatment for painful subacute thyroiditis is designed to provide symptomatic relief. Nonsteriodal anti-inflammatory agents can frequently be used to control mild thyroid pain. For more severe pain or significant thyrotoxicosis, high-dose glucocorticoids (prednisone 40 mg/day) can provide relief, and are usually tapered over 4–6 weeks.

## Suppurative thyroiditis

The thyroid gland is normally highly resistant to infection. This has been attributed to its location and encapsulation, high vascularity, high iodide content, the generation of hydrogen peroxide during synthesis of thyroid hormone, and extensive lymphatic drainage. Suppurative thyroiditis is most likely to occur in individuals with congenital anomalies such as a pyriform sinus fistula or persistent thyroglossal duct, those with pre-existing thyroid disease such as a degenerating thyroid nodule, or those who are otherwise immunocompromised or debilitated including individuals with acquired immunodeficiency syndrome (AIDS) or cancer.

Patients with suppurative bacterial thyroiditis usually present with fever, dysphagia, dysphonia, anterior neck pain, local lymphadenopathy, and have a tender erythematous thyroid mass. The patient is very uncomfortable and may sit with a flexed neck to avoid pressure on the thyroid. In children, suppurative thyroiditis affecting the left

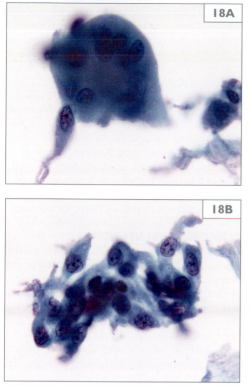

18 Subacute thyroiditis cytology. **A**: Giant cell; **B**: granuloma. (Courtesy of Dr. Tad Wieczorek.)

lobe of the thyroid is most commonly a result of direct extension from a pyriform sinus fistula (this tract rarely develops on the right), while a midline infection raises the possibility of a persistent thyroglossal duct. In adults, symptoms may not be as obvious as in children and they may instead present with a vague slightly painful mass in the thyroid region often without fever. This presentation is more common with fungal infections, parasitic infections, and mycobacterial thyroiditis. Fine-needle aspiration (FNA) under ultrasound guidance with Gram's stain and culture is the diagnostic test of choice when suppurative thyroiditis is suspected and may also provide therapeutic drainage. Treatment includes surgical drainage and appropriate antibiotics.

# Reidel's thyroiditis

Patients with Reidel's thyroiditis often present with a painless extremely hard, fixed goiter which is often described as 'rock-hard' or 'wood-like'; malignancy is often initially suspected. They may have dyspnea, hoarseness, aphonia, or dysphagia from tracheal or esophageal compression. Most patients are initially euthyroid at presentation and the disease may remain stable over many years or progress slowly to hypothyroidism. Hypoparathyroidism from fibrosis of adjacent parathyroid glands may also be present.

Open biopsy is usually required to diagnose Reidel's thyroiditis. The firmness of the gland and paucity of thyroid follicular cells often leads to an inadequate FNA biopsy. For this reason and to differentiate from the fibrotic changes associated with anaplastic thyroid carcinoma, surgical biopsy is preferred for diagnosis.

The management of Reidel's thyroiditis depends upon the clinical features of the disease and has been largely empiric. In more advanced cases, surgical intervention may be required to relieve compression. With less advanced disease, corticosteroids and tamoxifen have both been used successfully, either alone or in combination. Steroids may reduce inflammation and decrease the actions of fibrinogenic cytokines while it is believed that the response to tamoxifen is due to the inhibition of fibroblast proliferation by transforming growth factor (TGF)-beta as opposed to antiestrogen effects. Methotrexate is usually reserved for those with progressive Reidel's thyroiditis not responsive to other therapies. Since one-third of patients with Reidel's thyroiditis will develop an extracervical manifestation of multifocal fibrosclerosis such as retroperitoneal fibrosis, mediastinal fibrosis, or sclerosing cholangitis, screening for these other conditions should also be considered.

# Drug-induced thyroiditis

A number of drugs including amiodarone, interferon-alpha, lithium, and interleukin-2 (IL-2) can cause thyroiditis which may present with hypo- or hyperthyroidism. Interferon-alpha and IL-2 have both been associated with a painless lymphocytic thyroiditis. This is likely through an enhancement of underlying autoimmune processes as induction of, and increased anti-TPO antibody titers have been detected with exposure.

Lithium and amiodarone cause thyroid dysfunction via multiple different mechanisms. For example, amiodarone can cause iodine-induced disease or a destructive thyroiditis (*Table 4*). For differentiating between types 1 and 2 amiodarone-induced thyrotoxicosis, RAIU, IL-6 levels, and Doppler ultrasound for vascularity have all been proposed but in clinical practice it often remains difficult to distinguish between the two. As such, some clinicians treat for both concurrently using a combination of thionamide and steroids. Those with type 2 disease typically have a more rapid response to this strategy than those with type 1 disease, allowing tailoring of therapy to the underlying etiology based upon response. Thyroidectomy may be advisable for some patients.

## Thyroid nodules

### DEFINITION/OVERVIEW
Although the normal thyroid gland is fairly homogenous, nodules are not infrequent with about 5% of women and 1% of men in iodine-sufficient areas having palpable thyroid nodules. In autopsy series thyroid nodules are detected in 19–67% of the population, with higher frequencies noted in women and the elderly. The main clinical concern with thyroid nodules is that of thyroid cancer, which occurs in 5–10% of nodules, although it is estimated that only 1 in 15 cases of thyroid cancer are diagnosed premortem.

Approximately 1 in 10 to 1 in 20 solitary nodules are autonomous, with this being more common in Europe than the USA. Thyrotoxicity is related to the amount of autonomous tissue and is more common in nodules over 3 cm in diameter. In some individuals, multiple autonomous nodules may be present and such a toxic adenomatous goiter is sometimes referred to as Plummer's disease.

### CLINICAL PRESENTATION
Thyroid nodules are often asymptomatic and it is not unusual for them to go unrecognized by the patient, instead being noted by an acquaintance or family member, on routine examination, or incidentally on an unrelated radiologic study. When patients identify nodules themselves, it is often in the setting of increased awareness of the neck such as after a sore throat or cough. Occasionally, a painful, rapid expansion may be seen, which may be due to acute hemorrhage.

Large goiters, particularly those with substernal components, may cause venous congestion or tracheal compression (**19–24**). Patients may present with difficulty breathing,

**Table 4** Amiodarone-induced thyroid dysfunction

| | Type 1 | Type 2 | Hypothyroid |
|---|---|---|---|
| Mechanism | Iodine excess | Destructive thyroiditis | Iodine excess |
| Presentation | Thyrotoxicosis | Thyrotoxicosis | Hypothyroidism |
| Thyroid antibodies | Absent or present | Usually initially absent | Often present |
| RAI uptake | Low in iodine sufficient areas Variable in iodine deficient areas | <5 % | Low in iodine sufficient areas |
| Doppler ultrasound | Hypervascular | Reduced blood flow | Variable |
| IL-6 | Normal to mild elevation | Markedly elevated | Normal |
| Preferred treatment | Thionamides (possible potassium perchlorate and/or surgery) | Glucocorticoids | Levothyroxine |

**19** A man with retrosternal goiter causing venous congestion is shown (**A**). In (**B**) taken 6 months after resection, venous congestion has resolved. (From La Goitre by F. de Quervain, 1923.)

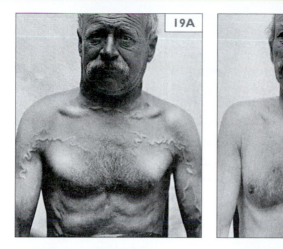

20 Goiter with multiple visible thyroid nodules is shown. (From La Goitre by F. de Quervain, 1923.)

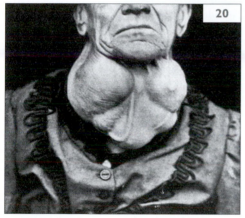

21 Large pendulous cystic nodule is shown. (From La Goitre by F. de Quervain, 1923.)

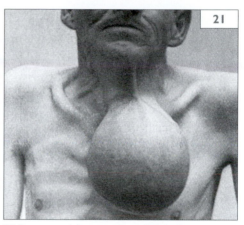

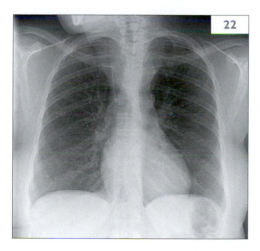

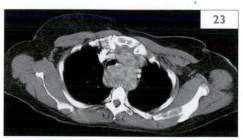

22, 23 Chest X-ray (**22**) and CT (**23**) are remarkable for large goiter with deviation of the trachea to the right. (Courtesy Dr. Sareh Parangi.)

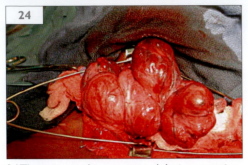

24 The goiter is shown exposed during resection. (Courtesy Dr. Sareh Parangi.)

particularly when lying flat, or experience a feeling of worsening of asthma symptoms. Patients with venous congestion may note facial fullness when they extend their arms above their head (Pemberton's sign) (**25**).

Patients with toxic adenomas may not have thyrotoxic symptoms at presentation. Those with symptomatic toxic adenomas tend to be older than individuals with Graves' disease and the onset of thyrotoxicosis is generally slower than in Graves' patients. When autonomy is longstanding, the normal thyroid tissue that surrounds the nodule is often atrophic.

### DIFFERENTIAL DIAGNOSIS

The differential of thyroid mass is quite broad as adenomas, carcinomas, thyroid cysts, hemiagenesis, thyroiditis, parathyroid lesions (including cysts, adenomas, and carcinomas), thyroid sarcoma, thyroid lymphoma, and metastatic cancer may also present as a thyroid mass on exam or ultrasound.

### DIAGNOSIS/INVESTIGATIONS

Current diagnostic algorithms in the evaluation of thyroid nodules focus on risk of malignancy, evidence of autonomy, and symptoms of compression or obstruction. Factors that increase the likelihood of thyroid malignancy include age younger than 20 or older than 60 years, prior exposure to ionizing radiation to the head or neck, family history of medullary or papillary thyroid cancer, and stigmata or family history of familial predisposing syndromes such as Gardner's syndrome (colonic polyps, osteomas,

soft tissue tumors), Carney complex (cardiac myxomas, spotty pigmentation), and Cowden's syndrome (hamartomas and neoplasia). Physical findings suggestive of malignancy include a hard, nontender nodule, fixed to adjacent tissue, and local lymphadenopathy.

Serum TSH should be measured in all patients with nodular disease. In most instances, serum TSH is normal and then further diagnostic evaluation is performed with ultrasound and FNA biopsy. If the TSH is low, isotopic scanning with $I^{131}$ or $I^{123}$ is often performed to determine if there is evidence of autonomy. Although not commonly performed, if the TSH is not suppressed but there is a high index of suspicion for autonomy, exogenous thyroid hormone can be administered prior to imaging to demonstrate nonsuppressibility (**26**). Nodules that exhibit evidence of autonomous function have a low risk of malignancy, although there have been reports of malignancy in autonomous nodules, particularly in those found to be follicular variant of papillary cancer.

Thyroid ultrasound can be used as an adjunct to physical examination for screening high-risk individuals (for example those with hereditary syndromes or prior radiation exposure), or for guidance of FNA. Ultrasonography more accurately detects the presence, location, and size of nodules within the thyroid gland than examination alone as 40–60% of thyroid nodules between 1 and 2 cm in diameter are not palpable on examination. Thyroid ultrasound can provide information including consistency, echogenicity, patterns of calcification, and Doppler blood flow. Nodules that are principally solid, hypoechoic, have irregular margins, contain microcalcifications, lack a halo, are taller than wide, or have increased vascular flow are of more concern for malignancy but ultrasound characteristics alone are usually not sensitive or specific enough for diagnostic purposes.

FNA biopsy is considered the most accurate test (diagnostic accuracy exceeding 90%) for the diagnosis of thyroid nodules. Biopsy is usually performed with a 27- or 25-gauge needle with sampling performed via capillary action or gentle aspiration, preferably under ultrasound guidance. Typical thyroid cytology findings include thyroid epithlial cells arranged in macrofollicles (**27A**) and microfollicles (**27B**). FNA results are usually categorized into one of

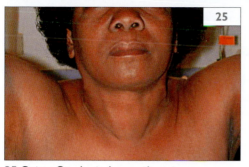

**25** Goiter. On physical exam there is venous engorgement with arms raised above the head (Pemberton's sign). (Courtesy of Dr. Sareh Parangi.)

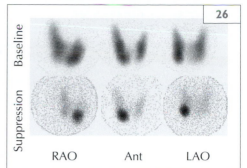

Baseline

Suppression

RAO          Ant          LAO

**26** Thyroid scintigraphy (suppression scan). RAO, anterior, and LAO views are shown. In the top panel, I$^{123}$ thyroid scintigraphy shows iodine uptake by the thyroid. In the lower panel, after treatment with exogenous thyroid hormone an autonomous area becomes apparent in the right inferior portion of the gland as the normal surrounding tissue is suppressed.

the following diagnostic categories: benign (negative), suspicious (indeterminate), malignant (positive), or unsatisfactory (nondiagnostic or insufficient). Although follicular neoplasm (microfollicular lesion) can be diagnosed by cytology, the distinction between follicular adenoma and carcinoma requires pathologic evaluation of a surgical specimen.

Since it is difficult to differentiate between thyroid and parathyroid tissue on FNA, if it is unclear on ultrasound if the area is a thyroid nodule or parathyroid adenoma, then a serum calcium should be checked and the aspirate evaluated for parathyroid hormone on washout. Parathyroid adenomas are typically extrathyroidal and hypoechoic on ultrasound. If the fluid removed from a cyst is clear and water-like then it may be a parathyroid cyst. The diagnosis can be confirmed by analyzing the fluid for parathyroid hormone level; although it is infrequent for parathyroid cysts to cause hyperparathyroidism, serum calcium should still be checked in this setting.

Although more expensive than ultrasound, computed tomography (CT) or magnetic resonance imaging (MRI) can be helpful in evaluating substernal goiters and defining the relationship of nodules to surrounding structures. This is most helpful if there is evidence of venous obstruction or difficulty breathing. Chest X-ray, barium swallow, and pulmonary functions tests with flow volume loop may also be used to determine the extent of obstruction.

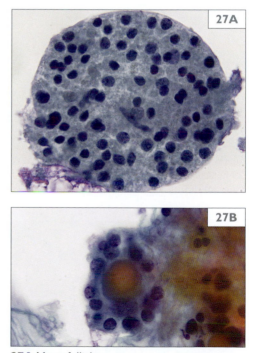

**27A** Macrofollicle.

**27B** Microfollicle.
(Both courtesy of Dr. Tad Wieczorek.)

## MANAGEMENT/TREATMENT

Nodules with malignant or indeterminate aspirates are usually treated surgically with the extent of surgery and follow-up therapy, if any, based upon the clinical situation. Various surgical specimens are shown in Figures 28–31. Obstructive goiters are generally treated surgically, although radioactive iodine treatment has been used in a limited fashion. Autonomous nodules without TSH suppression are often observed and may involute, stay the same, or grow. Once there is evidence of thyrotoxicosis, autonomous nodules are generally treated with radioiodine or surgery.

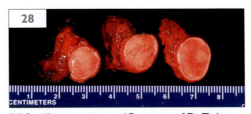

28 Papillary carcinoma. (Courtesy of Dr. Tad Wieczorek.)

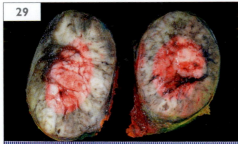

29 Follicular carcinoma. (Courtesy of Dr. Tad Wieczorek.)

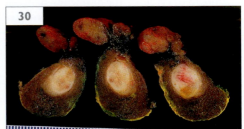

30 Follicular adenoma. (Courtesy of Dr. Tad Wieczorek.)

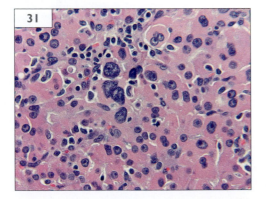

31 Anaplastic carcinoma histology. (Courtesy of Dr. Tad Wieczorek.)

# Thyroid cancer

### DEFINITION/OVERVIEW
There are approximately 30,000 new cases of thyroid cancer diagnosed yearly, about 2% of all malignancies, although this rate has been increasing due in part to more sensitive diagnostic methods resulting in earlier diagnosis. Fortunately, thyroid cancer is a very treatable disease, with only 1,500 disease-specific deaths occurring per year. Females are three times more likely to present with a thyroid nodule to be evaluated for cancer, but a thyroid nodule in a male is more suspicious for malignancy. A history of radiation exposure or positive family history, as well as physical examination findings, such as associated lymphadenopathy, also increase the likelihood of cancer. Even though most thyroid nodules encountered by clinicians will be benign, prompt work-up is necessary to ensure early and appropriate treatment can be instituted for those with malignancy.

### ETIOLOGY
The primary risk factors for thyroid carcinoma are a family history of thyroid cancer or related genetic syndromes and personal history of radiation exposure. In the 1940s and 1950s, low-dose irradiation was commonly used to treat acne, adenotonsillar hypertrophy, thymus enlargement, and other conditions. As reports of childhood thyroid cancer emerged, the practice was largely abandoned. Any patient with a history of radiation to the face, neck, or chest is at increased risk of developing thyroid neoplasms. Patients with this type of radiation exposure have up to a 50% chance of harboring cancer in a thyroid nodule and have a higher chance of cervical metastasis. The most common histology of postradiation thyroid cancer is papillary.

In 1986, reactor number four at the nuclear power plant in Chernobyl suffered a meltdown and explosion resulting in extensive radiation exposure to the surrounding area. Located in the northern part of what is now the Ukraine, Chernobyl is close to the Ukraine–Belarus border and Belarus actually received the majority of the fallout. In the months following the explosion, radioactivity was detected as far away as the United Kingdom. Local children exposed to the fallout had a 60-fold increase in thyroid carcinoma. A connection has been made between exposure to this disaster and a particular gene rearrangement (RET/PTC) in papillary thyroid cancers.

The full spectrum of genetic abnormalities resulting in thyroid cancer is actively being investigated. Certain familial syndromes such as Gardner's (autosomal dominant syndrome of colonic polyps, osteomas, and soft tissue tumors) and Cowden's (autosomal dominant syndrome of multiple hamartomas) are associated with well-differentiated thyroid cancer. The multiple endocrine neoplasia syndromes IIA and IIB are associated with medullary thyroid cancer.

### PATHOPHYSIOLOGY
The pathophysiology of thyroid cancer is influenced by the specific histologic diagnosis.

## Well differentiated thyroid cancer

### PAPILLARY THYROID CANCER
Papillary thyroid cancer (PTC) is the most common histology, accounting for 80% of all thyroid cancers. It has a bimodal distribution with peaks in the 20–30s and 50–60s. PTC has a propensity for lymphatic spread, and up to 80% of patients can present with microscopic disease in the lymph nodes. Indeed, the finding of cystic or calcified cervical lymph nodes should raise immediate suspicion for PTC. There is also a high incidence of multicentricity within the thyroid with up to 80% of thyroidectomy specimens demonstrating additional foci of PTC in the contralateral lobe.

Histologically, PTC is made of malignant epithelium usually forming papillae with characteristic nuclear clearing ('Orphan Annie eyes') and intranuclear inclusions and grooves (**32**). Concentric calcifications called psamomma bodies are seen in roughly half of specimens. Other histologic variations include follicular type, whose behavior is more similar to follicular cell carcinoma, a diffuse sclerosing type with a lack of papillae but many psamomma bodies, and the more clinically aggressive tall and columnar cell types.

Although there is no pathognomonic ultrasound findings, PTC are usually hypodense to surrounding thyroid tissue, and can be partially or entirely cystic (**33**). Microcalcifications, or eggshell-like peripheral calcifications, while present in some benign processes, increase with likelihood of PTC. FNA is highly sensitive and specific for PTC (**34**), and most patients will proceed to surgery knowing their diagnosis ahead of time (**35–40**) .

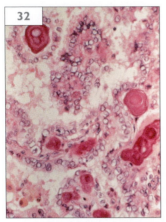

**32** Histology of papillary thyroid cancer demonstrating central nuclear clearing (Orphan Annie eyes) and psammoma bodies.

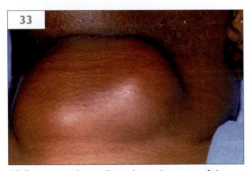

**33** Patient with papillary thyroid cancer of the thyroid isthmus presenting as an invasive anterior neck mass that is firm and minimally mobile on physical exam.

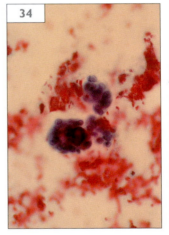

**34** Cytology from fine needle aspiration biopsy of a thyroid mass demonstrating papillary fronds consistent with papillary thyroid cancer.

**35** Surgical

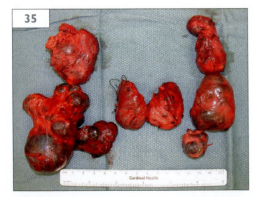

specimen of a total thyroidectomy (specimen in center) surrounded by bilateral neck dissections demonstrating metastatic papillary thyroid cancer that extensively involved both jugular lymph node chains. This demonstrates the potential for thyroid cancer to present primarily with cervical metastasis with minimal clinical changes in the thyroid gland.

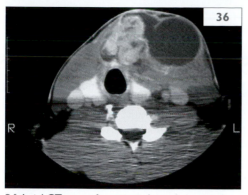

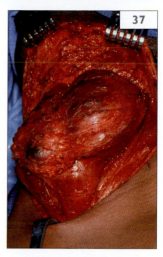

36 Axial CT scan of a patient demonstrating the growth pattern of papillary thyroid cancer arising from the isthmus and invading the strap muscles anteriorly.

37 Surgical findings of the patient in 36 demonstrating the growth pattern of papillary thyroid cancer arising from the isthmus and invading the strap muscles anteriorly. The picture is oriented with superior part of the neck at the top.

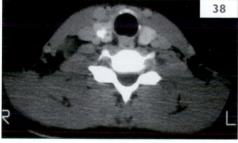

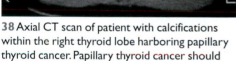

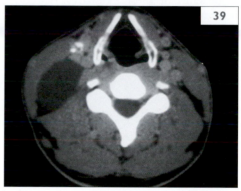

38 Axial CT scan of patient with calcifications within the right thyroid lobe harboring papillary thyroid cancer. Papillary thyroid cancer should always be considered in patients demonstrating calcifications within the thyroid gland on radiographic imaging.

39 CT scan of the patient in 38 at a higher axial plane in the neck. Findings include metastatic thyroid cancer to the right cervical region manifesting as a cystic neck mass as well as neck mass with calcifications. The differential diagnosis of any patient presenting with a cystic neck mass or lymph node with calcification should always include metastatic papillary thyroid cancer.

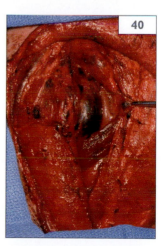

40 Intraoperative findings of the patient in 38 demonstrating the cystic neck mass just medial to the right sternocleidomastoid. The picture is oriented with the superior part of the neck at the top.

## Follicular cell cancer

In most regions, follicular cell carcinoma represents 5–15% of all thyroid cancers. This increases to 40% in areas that are endemic for goiter from iodine deficiency. The median age at diagnosis is 50. Follicular cancer tends to spread hematogenously, with 10–15% of patients presenting with systemic metastasis, with lung being the most common site, followed by bone, liver, brain, and other sites. These are iodine avid tumors, with three-quarters able to concentrate iodine.

For most follicular cancers, FNA can only make the diagnosis of a follicular lesion. The diagnosis of cancer relies on features detected during permanent sectioning, namely extracapsular spread or vascular invasion (**41**). If a follicular lesion presents with local extrathyroid spread or regional or distant metastasis, a preoperative diagnosis of follicular cancer can more assuredly be made. Minimally invasive follicular cancer is defined as those nodules with only capsular invasion, and is believed to be similar in prognosis and behavior to benign follicular adenomas. Moderately invasive follicular cancers are those demonstrating vascular invasion, and widely invasive are those with spread beyond their capsules.

## Hurthle cell cancer

Hurthle cell thyroid cancer is very similar to follicular cancer, and indeed may be a variant thereof. The hallmark is large, mitochondria-rich cells with eosinophilic cytoplasm. The presentation, reliance on permanent sectioning for diagnosis, and penchant for hematogenous spread are the same as follicular cancer. However, some authors believe Hurthle cell cancer to be a more aggressive entity, demonstrating up to one-third as multicentric and one-quarter with lymph node spread at diagnosis. Hurthle cell cancers are less iodine avid than follicular cancers, but they do tend to produce thyroglobulin.

## Insular thyroid cancer

This rare disease entity is distinguished by the identification of small clusters of malignant cells similar in appearance to pancreatic islet cells. Insular thyroid cancer can occur in association with papillary or follicular cancer or as an independent process. Insular carcinoma arising independently is associated with a more aggressive clinical course. These lesions are typically iodine avid.

### Medullary thyroid cancer

Medullary thyroid cancer (MTC) arises from the parafollicular C cells of neural crest origin. Approximately two-thirds arise spontaneously, usually as a solitary nodule in patients in their sixth or seventh decade, with equal distribution between females and males. The remaining third are associated with familial autosomal dominant mutations of the RET proto-oncogene, either in isolation or as part of the syndromes of multiple endocrine neoplasia (MEN) 2A and 2B. Familial MTC is associated with multicentricity.

Measurement of serum calcitonin can be useful in the diagnosis of MTC, and can be used for postoperative monitoring for recurrence. Up to half of patients will present with local or distant disease; the favored sites of spread being cervical lymph nodes, then mediastinum, lung, liver, and bone. Some patients may present with pain from local invasion. The overall clinical behavior is more aggressive than the differentiated thyroid cancers above, but less aggressive than anaplastic cancer.

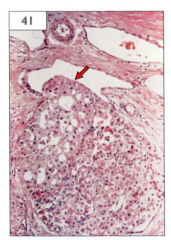

**41** Histology of follicular adenocarcinoma of the thyroid demonstrating angioinvasion (arrow).

## Anaplastic thyroid cancer

Anaplastic thyroid cancer is an uncommon entity, accounting for less than 2% of thyroid cancers, but causing the most deaths. The prognosis is grim, with fewer than 10% of patients surviving beyond 5 years, and most patients only surviving 3–6 months after diagnosis. The typical presentation is a female in her 50s or 60s with a rapidly enlarging thyroid mass. Half of patients present with metastatic disease, primarily mediastinum and lung, followed by bone and brain (**42, 43**).

Respiratory symptoms are common, and airway management with a tracheotomy is often necessary. In some patients, extensive tracheal invasion requires endoluminal stenting to alleviate asphyxiation. Anaplastic cancer is believed to be on the far end of a spectrum of dedifferentiation of thyroid cells, as evidenced by common genetic alterations, especially with papillary cancer. Most anaplastic cancers have lost their ability to concentrate iodine or elaborate thyroglobulin.

## Thyroid lymphoma

Primary thyroid lymphoma is uncommon, accounting for approximately 2% of thyroid malignancies. Many patients have a history of autoimmune thyroiditis, particularly Hashimoto's, and 85% of thyroid lymphoma specimens have thyroiditis features present histologically. A typical presentation is enlargement of a previously existing goiter, or as a rapidly enlarging thyroid or cervical mass. 'B' symptoms such as fever, weight loss, and night sweats can also be present.

Thyroid lymphomas are typically nonHodgkin's lymphomas of the B-cell type, though T cell lymphomas can occur, particularly in human T-lymphotrophic virus (HTLV)-endemic areas. Many patients have laboratory evidence of longstanding hypothyroidism, with elevated TSH and antithyroid peroxidase or thyroglobulin antibodies. Elevated immunoglobulins or LDH can also be seen. Traditionally, an incisional or excisional biopsy was needed to establish the diagnosis accurately, sent fresh for lymphoma work-up. However, advances in flow cytometry have made diagnosis by FNA more reliable when performed by experienced clinicians.

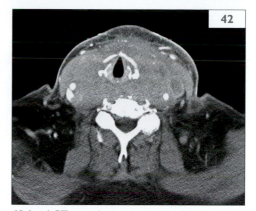

**42** Axial CT scan demonstrating invasive anaplastic thyroid cancer invading the larynx and encasing the great vessels.

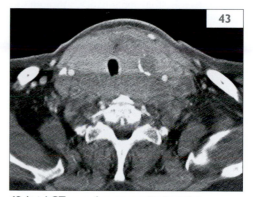

**43** Axial CT scan demonstrating invasive anaplastic thyroid cancer encasing the tracheal airway.

## CLINICAL PRESENTATION

The first discovery of a thyroid nodule is often made on physical examination or is an incidental finding on imaging work-up for another reason. Thyroid nodules are not uncommon, with studies reporting 30–50% of individuals harboring incidental nodules. The vast majority of nodules will be benign, with less than 10% representing malignancy. Certain features of the history and physical exam may suggest a malignancy. As mentioned above, patients with a history of radiation exposure or family history are at increased risk. In addition, a history of a rapidly enlarging mass is more suspicious for malignancy (**33**); however, a rapidly enlarging, painful thyroid mass may represent hemorrhage into a benign cyst. More aggressive thyroid cancers can manifest early with respiratory symptoms, due either to airway compression, invasion of the trachea, or compression or invasion of the recurrent laryngeal nerves leading to vocal cord dysfunction.

Most patients presenting with thyroid cancer are euthyroid. Symptoms of hyper- or hypothyroidism do not rule out cancer but may prompt further work-up for a benign cause.

Nodules that are greater than 1 cm can usually be palpated. Fixation to surrounding structures and palpable cervical lymphadenopathy increase the suspicion for malignancy, though in particular lymphadenopathy can occur in benign processes such as Graves' and Hashimoto's. History and physical examination findings that are more indicative of a malignant process are summarized in *Table* 5. Well-differentiated thyroid cancers (papillary, follicular, and Hurthle cell) can be staged using one of four grading systems: AJCC, AGES, AMES, or MACIS. Again, depending on the histology, cancer of the thyroid has many different presentations and behaviors, outlined above.

## DIFFERENTIAL DIAGNOSIS

The primary differential diagnosis is between benign and malignant processes. Thyroid cancer typically presents as a nodule, and may not be able to be distinguished from a benign adenoma without surgical excision. Metastases from renal cell, melanoma, breast, and lung cancer can also present as thyroid nodules. Multinodular goiters usually represent benign processes, but large or suspicious nodules must be investigated independently as they carry the same risk for carcinoma. Diffuse thyroid enlargement may be benign goiter, an inflammatory or infectious process, or neoplastic infiltration.

## DIAGNOSIS

Palpation of the thyroid, appreciating the overall size and consistency of the thyroid as well as the character of any nodules is the first step in diagnosis. Tenderness, fixation to surrounding structures, and associated cervical lymphadenopathy should be appreciated (*Table* 5). A screening TSH can be ordered to evaluate for functional nodules. FNA is the mainstay of the work-up for a thyroid nodule. A 27-gauge needle loaded on a syringe is inserted into a palpable nodule while gentle suction is maintained with backpressure on the syringe plunger. Several passes are made in different directions taking care to stay within the nodule. The hub of the needle is watched for return of serous material. Aspiration of blood decreases the interpretability of the FNA, and if this occurs the needle should be taken out, pressure should be held, and the FNA should be reattempted with a fresh needle. Multiple samples should be taken, and spread amongst slides for both air dry and cytologic fixation. Involvement of experienced clinicians in the process of FNA increases the diagnostic yield. If the nodule is found to be cystic and fluid-filled, the fluid should be sent for cytology. Bloody fluid may represent hemorrhage into a

---

**Table 5 History and physical examination findings suggestive of thyroid cancer**

**History**

Family history of multiple endocrine neoplasia, or medullary thyroid cancer

Personal history of head and neck irradiation or radiation exposure

Symptoms of airway compression or voice changes

Symptoms of hemoptysis

Rapid tumor growth

**Physical examination**

Very firm or hard nodule

Fixation of nodule to surrounding structures

Regional lymphadenopathy including cystic neck mass

Distant metastases

Large nodule (>4 cm)

cyst or carcinoma. If a lesion is found on imaging to have both solid and cystic components, an attempt should be made to sample the solid component.

As mentioned above, FNA is highly sensitive and specific when diagnosing PTC. Follicular and Hurthle cell nodules cannot be distinguished between benign and malignant on FNA alone. Anaplastic cancer and thyroid lymphoma may require additional tissue from an incisional biopsy to make the diagnosis accurately. Nondiagnostic FNA should never be interpreted as negative for cancer.

Ultrasonography is very useful for evaluating the thyroid. It can detect additional nonpalpable nodes or differentiate between nodules and lobar hypertrophy. Certain characteristics of nodules, such as calcifications or cystic components, can increase the suspicion for cancer. Ultrasound can also be used to evaluate regional lymphatics, and can be used to guide FNA for nonpalpable nodules or for sampling the solid component of a cystic nodule.

CT and MRI scans of the thyroid usually do not add much to the work-up of thyroid cancer. For patients with well-differentiated thyroid cancers who are being considered for postoperative radioactive iodine therapy (see below), use of CT with iodinated contrast media is contraindicated because it delays treatment for up to 3 months. If imaging must be obtained in these patients, such as for suspicion of tracheal invasion or to evaluate substernal extension, MRI is preferred. Postoperatively, MRI is also better at distinguishing recurrent disease from postoperative fibrosis. In patients who present with massive, rapidly enlarging goiters suspicious for anaplastic carcinoma or lymphoma where tissue diagnosis or airway management is needed, a CT with contrast is appropriate for surgical planning.

Radionucleotide scanning with radioactive iodine is useful for assessing the functionality of a nodule, but is not useful in determining risk for cancer. Nodules that fail to take up iodine on scan are referred to as cold nodules. Traditionally, cold nodules have been considered higher risk for cancer. However, the majority of patient with thyroid nodules are cold on scan making radionucleotide ineffective in screening for cancer risk. Additionally,

hyperfunctional or hot nodules have been traditionally considered to be benign but numerous cases have been reported of hot nodules harboring thyroid cancer. The primary role of radionucleotide scanning is for ablation and post-treatment surveillance.

## MANAGEMENT/TREATMENT

Surgery is the primary treatment for most thyroid cancer. For some well-differentiated thyroid nodules, there is controversy regarding the extent of surgical resection (lobectomy versus subtotal or total thyroidectomy). However, the basic guiding principles are as follows:

- If a patient has no worrisome risk factors and a favorable histology (e.g. a young woman with an isolated 1.0 papillary cancer with no extracapsular spread) a lobectomy may be appropriate and spares the patient a lifetime of thyroid hormone replacement.
- If unfavorable features are seen in permanent histology after a lobectomy, such as vascular invasion or diffuse infiltration of the thyroid, removal of the contralateral lobe is indicated.
- If there is high suspicion for multicentricity (e.g. large papillary thyroid cancers and familial medullary thyroid cancer), or at least some disease in the contralateral lobe, an upfront total thyroidectomy is indicated or removal of contralateral lobe after unilateral lobectomy.
- If postoperative radioactive iodine is planned for aggressive histology or known extrathyroid disease, a total thyroidectomy permits more effective detection and treatment of residual local and distant microscopic disease (see below).

The standard surgical approach is through a small horizontal incision just above the clavicle. The strap muscles are divided in the midline down to the gland. One lobe is removed at a time if both are being taken, with care to preserve the parathyroid glands and recurrent laryngeal nerves.

In patients with clinically apparent nodal disease in the central compartment or lateral cervical lymph node chains, a neck dissection is obviously warranted to remove gross disease. En bloc lymphadenectomy is preferred in these situations over removal of individual nodes given the high incidence of microscopic disease. The role of neck dissection in the clinically negative neck is more controversial.

Radioactive iodine ($^{131}$I) has proven a very effective treatment for microscopic and distant disease in well-differentiated thyroid cancer (i.e. cancers able to uptake and concentrate the radioiodine). The typical sequence of treatment is total thyroidectomy, followed by a 4–6-week period of thyroid withdrawal during which time the TSH level is allowed to rise to greater than 30 µIU/mL. Then, while maximal stimulation of any remaining thyroid tissue is occurring, whole body radioiodine scanning is performed, followed the next day by $^{131}$I ablation (**44**).

After ablation, the patient is started on thyroid suppression therapy with levothyroxine to maintain a low level of TSH through feedback mechanisms on the hypothalamus. The target level of TSH is determined by the aggressiveness of the cancer, with lower or undetectable levels desired for higher-risk patients. Serum thyroglobulin (Tg) is followed for recurrence. An important exception to this is patients with antithyroglobulin (anti-Tg) antibodies, in whom Tg levels cannot be followed. In these patients, the level of anti-Tg has been shown somewhat to correlate with recurrence.

In contrast to patients with well-differentiated thyroid cancer, for patients with anaplastic cancer or thyroid lymphoma, chemotherapy and radiation are the primary treatment modalities, and there is no role for radioactive iodine. For lymphoma, the treatment regimen is driven by the specific types of cells involved, but the most common for non-Hodgkin's lymphoma is a combination of cyclophosphamide, doxorubicin, and vincristine in combination with radiotherapy. Treatment for anaplastic cancer is largely experimental, with some combination of chemotherapy, external beam radiation, and surgical debulking performed as much for palliation as curative intent. The main role of surgery in both anaplastic cancer and thyroid lymphoma is obtaining tissue for diagnosis and airway management with tracheotomy.

Patients with a family history of medullary thyroid cancer who are positive for the RET mutation often undergo prophylactic thyroidectomy at a young age. Total thyroidectomy with central compartment neck dissection is the minimum treatment for any patient presenting with clinically evident MTC. Further neck dissection is based on clinical findings.

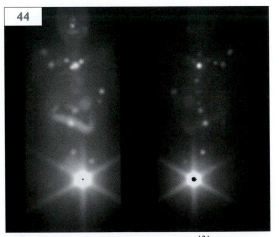

**44** Radioactive iodine uptake scan with I$^{131}$ demonstrating metastatic papillary thyroid cancer. The large starburst pattern in the lower part of the image is consistent with metastasis to the pelvic bone.

# Diabetes mellitus

Amit Dayal

Mary Ann Emanuele

Nicholas Emanuele

**Introduction**

**Retinopathy**

**Nephropathy**

**Neuropathy**

**Skin manifestations**

**The diabetic foot**

**Cardiovascular disease in diabetes**

**Secondary causes of diabetes**

**Therapeutic options for type 2 diabetes**

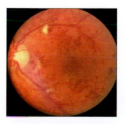
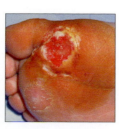
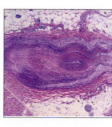
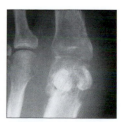

## Introduction

Diabetes mellitus (DM) is a disease which afflicts more than 20 million people in the United States (US) and many more world-wide. Projected figures are that the number of individuals with diabetes will increase from 166 million in 2000 to 330 million by 2030; areas most affected by this increase include Africa, the eastern Mediterranean region, and southeast Asia where a quadrupling of the incidence of DM is expected to occur. In the US, the lifetime risk for developing diabetes in an individual born after 2000 is 33% for Caucasians and 50% for Hispanics. These numbers reflect the explosion of obesity in the US and worldwide. Type 1 diabetes, accounting for about 10% of people with diabetes mellitus, is an autoimmune disease wherein the insulin-producing β cells of the pancreas are destroyed. Treatment relies solely on the use of insulin.

Type 2 diabetes mellitus, seen in almost 90% of the diabetic population, has two pathophysiologic loci, insulin resistance and relative or absolute hypoinsulinemia. Insulin resistance, in addition to participating in the development of hyperglycemia, can also lead to hypertriglyceridemia, low levels of high-density lipoprotein (HDL)-cholesterol, hypertension, and truncal obesity and this constellation of features is commonly referred to as the metabolic syndrome. The treatment of type 2 diabetes initially relies on the use of oral agents and subcutaneously injected medications which augment insulin secretion, reduce excessively high glucagon levels, decrease insulin resistance, or interrupt intestinal carbohydrate absorption. These agents may be used in combination with a variety of insulins as pancreatic function wanes.

# Retinopathy

### DEFINITION/OVERVIEW
Retinopathy is the most common microvascular complication of diabetes and accounts for 10,000 cases of new blindness per year. This complication is seen in both types 1 and 2 diabetes, but the onset of type 2 diabetes is insidious and it may develop many years before diagnosis. There is evidence that retinopathy may begin to develop 7 years before the clinical diagnosis of type 2 diabetes is made. Retinopathy is known to initially worsen, and then improve as better glycemic control is instituted. It may also progress with pregnancy, with improvement after delivery.

### ETIOLOGY
The major mechanism for the development of retinopathy is chronic hyperglycemia. Accumulation of polyols and advanced glycosylation end-products, oxidative stress, and protein kinase C activation may mediate the effects of hyperglycemia. Excessive levels of intraocular vascular endothelial growth factor, a deficiency of pigment epithelium-derived factor (a protein that inhibits neovascularization), and reduced concentrations of transforming growth factor-$\beta$ (a protein that may inhibit endothelial proliferation) may play a role. Insulin-like growth factor-1 (IGF-1) seems to be permissive in the development of retinopathy. In addition to these chemical factors, genetic factors seem to play a role as genetic clustering of retinopathy has been reported.

### PATHOPHYSIOLOGY
Diabetic retinopathy may be divided into preproliferative (or background) retinopathy, and the more serious proliferative retinopathy. First, there is the preproliferative phase. Because of the alterations described in Etiology (above), there is loss of the vascular supporting cells, the pericytes, which allows the development of microaneurisms, small out-pouching from the capillaries of the retina, as well as dot intraretinal hemorrhages (**45, 46**). There may be a progressive increase in the number of hemorrhages as well as the development of cotton wool spots, both manifestations of regional ischemia due to microvascular disease.

Proliferative retinopathy develops because of the formation of new blood vessels, the process of neovascularization (**46**). This is likely due, at least in part, to the growth factor imbalance described, as well as to loss of pericytes, which may have a contractile function regulating retinal blood flow. This dysregulation may lead

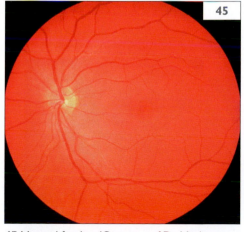

**45** Normal fundus. (Courtesy of Dr. Mark Dailey.)

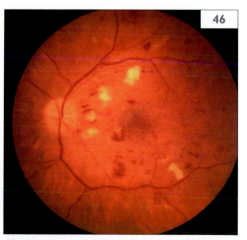

**46** Microaneurisms, flame hemorrhages, cotton wool spots, and neovascularization of the disc. (Courtesy of Dr. Mark Dailey.)

to ischemia, an additional stimulus to neovascularization. The new and fragile blood vessels grow into the vitreous where they may burst, with the vitreous hemorrhage causing visual loss (**47**). Scarring in the hemorrhage attaching to the retina can then retract causing retinal detachment and more visual problems.

Excess vascular endothelial growth factor (VEGF) may cause disruption of the blood–retinal barrier. This can lead to macular edema which may result is substantial central visual loss. When the fluid elements of this macular edema reabsorb, the lipid and lipoprotein elements remaining cause hard exudates (**48**).

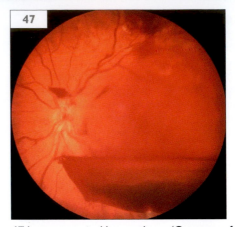

47 Large preretinal hemorrhage. (Courtesy of Dr. Mark Dailey.)

### CLINICAL PRESENTATION
There is a progression from microaneurisms and dot hemorrhages to neovascularization (**45, 46, 48**). After neovascularization, its attendant problems, vitreous hemorrhage, retinal detachment, and glaucoma may follow (**47**). Macular edema can occur anywhere during the course of this progression.

### DIAGNOSIS
The traditional method of detection of diabetic retinopathy is by ophthalmoscopic physical examination, preferably through dilated pupils. However, a variety of photographic techniques may complement the physical examination or even replace it. Fluorescein angiography is a useful method for characterization of the retinal vasculature (**49**).

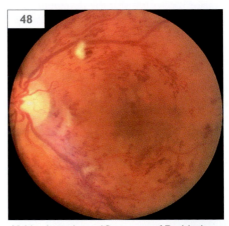

48 Hard exudates. (Courtesy of Dr. Mark Dailey.)

### MANAGEMENT/TREATMENT
Observational as well as interventional studies have shown that maintenance of good glycemic control is of ocular benefit. Several prospective trials have documented the importance of good blood pressure control in ocular protection and, in fact, there was a 47% reduced risk in deterioration in visual acuity in the United Kingdom Prospective Diabetes Study.

In addition, several eye-specific treatments are effective. Panretinal scatter photocoagulation benefits people with proliferative retinopathy or neovascular glaucoma. Focal photocoagulation may be used for macular edema. Vitrectomy can be used for nonclearing vitreous hemorrhage or traction detachment of the retina. Novel approaches, such as blockade of VEGF, are being tested.

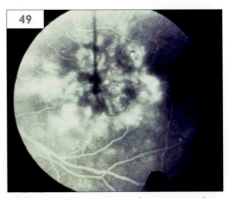

49 Fluorescein angiogram showing vascular leakage. (Courtesy of Dr. Mark Dailey.)

# Nephropathy

## DEFINITION/OVERVIEW

Diabetic nephropathy is the leading cause of renal failure in individuals on dialysis. It has been generally defined as the presence of more than 500 mg albumin in a 24-hour urine collection. This is overt nephropathy. However, patients first go through stages of lesser protein spillage, termed microalbuminuria. Proteinuria occurs in 15–40% of individuals with type 1 diabetes, the prevalence peaking at 15–20 years of diabetes duration. The prevalence varies from 5–20% in patients with type 2 diabetes.

## ETIOLOGY

At most, probably no more that 40% of diabetic people develop nephropathy. It is clear that there is familial clustering of this complication, and, thus, genetic susceptibility plays a role in the development of nephropathy in both type 1 and type 2 diabetes. Given this background, there are several modifiable factors that lead to the clinical initiation and progression of nephropathy including hyperglycemia and hypertension. Other etiological factors include glomerular hyperfiltration, proteinuria itself, smoking, dyslipidemia, and dietary factors including protein and fat.

## PATHOPHYSIOLOGY

The classic histologic changes of diabetic nephropathy are increased glomerular basement membrane (GBM) width and mesangial expansion (**50, 51**). Not only is the GBM thickened, but it is biochemically and functionally defective, allowing albumin leakage into the urine. The defective function of the GBM coupled with increased transglomerular pressure (caused by excessive constriction of the efferent glomerular arteriole compared to the afferent arteriole) leads to proteinuria. The expansion of the mesangium decreases glomerular capillary luminal space and, thus, reduces glomerular filtration.

The mechanistic role of hyperglycemia in the pathophysiology is complex and is mediated through increases in growth factors (such as transforming growth factor-β and VEGF), activation of protein kinase C, increase in oxidative stress, enhanced formation of advanced glycosylation end-products, and increased flux through the aldose reductase pathway.

## CLINICAL PRESENTATION

If untreated, patients first present with no evidence of renal disease but then progress from microalbuminuria to nephropathy to nephrotic syndrome and, finally, to dialysis-requiring end-stage renal disease.

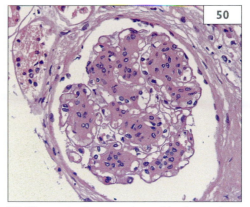

**50** Glomerulus from a patient with advanced diabetic nephropathy stained with PAS. Nodular mesangial expansion is seen (Kimmelstiel–Wilson nodules). (Courtesy of Dr. Maria Picken.)

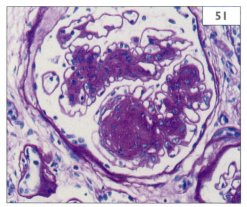

**51** Glomerulus from a patient with advanced diabetic nephropathy stained with HE. Nodular mesangial expansion is seen (Kimmelstiel–Wilson nodules). (Courtesy of Dr. Maria Picken.)

## DIFFERENTIAL DIAGNOSIS

In diabetic patients with impaired renal function and/or proteinuria, symptoms of urinary tract obstruction and systemic diseases other than diabetes (such as lupus or hepatitis B or C among others) should be sought. Imaging or biopsy may be considered in selected cases.

## DIAGNOSIS

The diagnosis is easily made in long-term (>10 years) type 1 diabetic people with renal functional impairment and proteinuria, especially if there is concurrent retinopathy, the retinal–renal syndrome. The diagnosis may be less certain in people with type 2 diabetes, since the actual time of onset of the disease is often not clear and about one in four patients may not have retinopathy.

Screening for proteinuria can be done with a 24-hour or shorter, timed urine collection, but is much more conveniently accomplished with a spot urine sample. Because of the well-known variability in day-to-day urinary albumin excretion, the diagnosis should only be made if two of three specimens collected over a 3–6 month period are abnormal. An additional diagnostic caveat is that the presence of factors other than renal disease, which can elevate urinary albumin excretion, must be ruled out. These include urinary tract infection, hematuria, acute febrile illness, uncontrolled hypertension, heart failure, vigorous exercise, and short-term pronounced hyperglycemia.

## MANAGEMENT/TREATMENT

Good glycemic control has been shown to protect kidney function and is a major part of therapy. Equally important is blood pressure control. The goal is a blood pressure less than 130/80 (<125/75 if serum creatinine is elevated and proteinuria is >1 g/24 hours). Therapy should be initiated with angiotensin-converting enzyme (ACE) inhibitors or angiotensin receptor blockers, but many patients will need three to four different agents to achieve goals. There are early data suggesting that statin therapy may preserve kidney function, as may dietary protein restriction.

# Neuropathy

### DEFINITION/OVERVIEW
Diabetic neuropathy can be subdivided into generalized symmetric polyneuropathies and focal/multifocal mononeuropathies. Symmetric polyneuropathies include three distinct entities: acute sensory, chronic sensorimotor, and autonomic neuropathies. Focal/multifocal neuropathies are further subcategorized into cranial, truncal, focal limb, and diabetic amyotrophy. Chronic distal sensorimotor polyneuropathy (DPN) and autonomic neuropathy (AN) are the two most common forms. A simple definition of DPN is 'the presence of symptoms and/or signs of peripheral nerve dysfunction in people with diabetes after the exclusion of other causes'. DPN is the most common form of neuropathy, but is subclinical in about half of cases. AN may manifest itself in one or multiple organ systems. More than 50% of all diabetics may expect to develop a diabetic neuropathy. The duration of diabetes correlates well with the development of neuropathy. Type 1 diabetics typically begin to develop neuropathies after 5 years, while in type 2 diabetics the neuropathy may begin prior to the clinical diagnosis of diabetes.

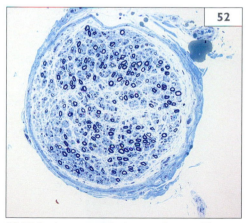

**52** Diabetic neuropathy in a sural nerve. Note the wedge-shaped areas with axonal loss and a mild overall decrease in axonal number. (Courtesy of Dr. Henry Brown.)

### ETIOLOGY
The duration of diabetes, as well as the level of hyperglycemia plays a central role in the development of diabetic neuropathies. Other factors thought to play a role in the development of neuropathy include hypertension, hyperlipidemia, obesity, tobacco use and alcohol consumption. Acute sensorimotor neuropathy, although rare, is thought to be a result of marked metabolic derangement including ketoacidosis and rapid fluctuations in glycemic control. Mononeuropathies have two distinct etiologies. The most common form is entrapment. This can be seen in up to 30% of diabetic people. Microvascular infarcts, whose symptoms are self-limiting, also lead to mononeuropathies and are rare in comparison.

### PATHOPHYSIOLOGY
Hyperglycemia in DPN and AN leads to the intracellular accumulation of sorbitol, via the actions of the aldose reductase pathway. As a result, cellular osmolality is increased and myoinostitol is decreased. Hyperglycemia also leads to the development of advanced glycosylation end-products. These factors, coupled with the increased development of reactive oxygen species (multiple pathways) and the decrease in available antioxidants, leads to a functional limitation in axonal transport, impairment of neurotropism, and alteration of gene expression. Ischemia is also thought to play a role in the development of polyneuropathies. Heightened expression of protein kinase C (PKC), PAI-1, TGF-B and VEGF in diabetes leads to increase in endothelial injury and micro/macrovascular occlusion. An example of diabetic neuronal loss in a sural nerve biopsy is shown in Figure **52**.

### CLINICAL PRESENTATION
DPN most frequently presents as a parasthesia, hyperesthesia, deep aching pain, burning, or electrical sensation. These symptoms are typically worse at night. It is symmetric in distribution. The disease typically affects the distal extremities; most commonly the feet and lower legs. It has a progressive symmetric distal to proximal course, leading to the classic stocking-glove distribution. In 50% of instances, DPN is subclinical and may present

with calluses or a painless foot ulcer. Acute sensorimotor neuropathy presents with similar findings as DPN. The hallmark is the sudden onset, severity, and typical self-limiting course.

ANs present in a variety of ways, dependent upon the organ systems that are affected. Cardiac AN may present as decreased exercise tolerance, fatigue, weakness with exercise, postural hypotension, dizziness, tachycardia, or overt syncope. In many instances, cardiac AN is silent. Esophageal motility disturbances are not uncommon. These are manifested by either excessive peristaltic contractions (**53**) or absent contractions (**54**). Gastric presentation of AN is varied. It ranges from gastroparesis, abdominal pain, vomiting, belching, early satiety, and constipation to diarrhea and incontinence. Genitourinary symptoms include vaginal dryness, erectile dysfunction, nocturia, urinary retention, urinary incontinence or increased urinary frequency; striking examples of neurogenic bladders are shown in Figures **55** and **56**. Sudomotor symptoms associated with AN include hyperhydrosis, anhydrosis, heat intolerance, and dry skin.

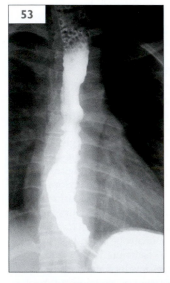

**53** Tertiary contractions in the esophagus from a diabetic patient. (Courtesy of Dr. Laurie Lomasney.)

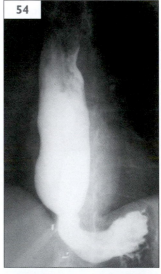

**54** Absence of contractions in the esophagus from a diabetic patient. (Courtesy of Dr. Laurie Lomasney.)

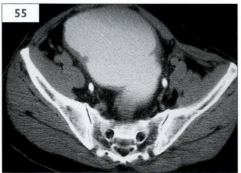

**55** Neurogenic bladder. (Courtesy of Dr. Laurie Lomasney.)

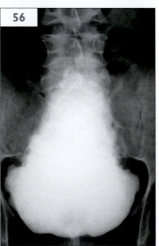

**56** Neurogenic bladder with diverticuli. (Courtesy of Dr. Laurie Lomasney.)

Focal/multifocal mononeuropathies also have a varied presentation. Patients with diabetic amyotrophy will present with unilateral or bilateral severe neuropathic pain. Physical findings include proximal thigh weakness and atrophy. Those with thoracic polyradiculopathy may present with severe pain in a band-like distribution about the chest or abdomen. Cranial mononeuropathies can affect the oculomotor, trochlear, and abducens nerves, leading to ophthalmoplegia. Patients with diabetic ophthalmoplegia present with unilateral pain, ptosis, and diplopia. Peripheral mononeuropathies may produce effects in the median, ulnar, radial, and peroneal nerves. This has an acute onset and may result in symptoms such as foot drop.

## DIFFERENTIAL DIAGNOSIS

Chronic inflammatory demyelinating process (CIDP), $B_{12}$ deficiency, spinal stenosis, hypothyroidism, and uremia occur more frequently in the diabetic population. The use of imaging, laboratory work-up and neurology referral should be used to elucidate the etiology of the neuropathy. In asymmetric polyneuro-pathies, the diagnosis of systemic vasculitus should be entertained.

## DIAGNOSIS

DPN is a clinical diagnosis and a complete history and physical examination is essential. Simple inspection of the feet may reveal calluses or ulcerations of an insensate foot. Regularly checking pinprick, temperature perception, vibratory sense (using a 128 Hz tuning fork), pressure sensation (using a 10 g monofilament), and ankle reflexes is recommended. The combination of any two positive tests has 87% sensitivity for detecting DPN. Detection of AN involves diverse testing based on the organ system involved, but details are beyond the scope of this chapter. Focal/multifocal neuropathies can be diagnosed through meticulous history and physical examination. Electrophysiological studies may aid in the determination of the site of nerve entrapment or infarction.

## MANAGEMENT/TREATMENT

There are numerous drugs used to treat DPN. The first goal of therapy, (with all neuropathies), should be to improve glycemic control. Regular inspection of the feet may prevent amputation by identifying early foot lesions otherwise missed because of insensate feet. Subsequent therapy should be directed at appropriately controlling blood pressure and following cholesterol guidelines. Medications for symptomatic relief of pain include tricyclic drugs (e.g. amitryptilline), anticonvulsants (gabapentin and topiramate), pregabalin, capsaicin cream, selective serotonin reuptake inhibitors (SSRI), and duloxetine. Vasodilators have been shown to have limited success. For refractory pain, the use of opioids or pain service consultation may be necessary. Treatment of mononeuropathies may include surgical decompression of entrapped nerves.

Cardiac AN may respond to beta-blockers, ACE inhibitors and supervised exercise therapy. Postural hypotension, after exclusion of other diseases, may respond to the use of midodrine or octreotide. Gastroparesis, chronic abdominal pain, and vomiting may respond to frequent small meals, prokinetic agents (metoclopro-mide, erythromycin), gastric pacing, pyloric botox, or enteral feedings. Constipation may be approached with high fiber diets, bulking agents, and osmotic laxatives. Erectile dysfunction may respond to phosphodiesterase-5 inhibitors (sildenafil, vardenafil, and tadalafil), prostaglandins, or a prosthesis. Bladder dysfunction can be treated with bethanecol or intermittent catheterization.

# Skin manifestations

### OVERVIEW
Skin manifestations in diabetes mellitus are common. Many skin manifestations seen in association with diabetes mellitus may also be seen in other conditions. These lesions may result from microangiopathy, hyperinsulinemia, hyperlipidemia, reaction to treatments, or immune compromise leading to infections.

## Necrobiosis lipoidica diabeticorum

### DEFINITION/OVERVIEW
This disease is an uncommon finding affecting 0.3–1.2% of patients. Necrobiosis is most commonly seen in type 1 diabetic individuals, although it manifests in those with type 2 diabetes and patients with insulin resistance. About one in four patients with necrobiosis do not carry a diagnosis of diabetes. Females are three times more likely to develop these lesions.

### ETIOLOGY
This skin lesion may be the result of diabetic microangiopathy, immune complex disease, abnormal production of collagen, and impaired neutrophil migration. The lesions are commonly associated with poor glycemic control, but there is no evidence that necrobiosis is prevented by good glycemic control.

### PATHOPHYSIOLOGY
Biopsy examination of necrobiosis reveals thinning central dermis, collagen degeneration, and granulomatous inflammation of the subcutaneous tissue as well as blood vessel wall thickening.

### CLINICAL PRESENTATION
The lesions are most common on the pretibial aspect of the leg, and are generally bilateral in presentation (**57**). Less often they are found on the trunk, arms, and face. Initially they are seen as small red papules. These eventually coalesce to form a large circular lesion with a waxy yellow center. Telangiectasias are seen in this area of the lesion (**58**). Mature lesions have been characterized as having a 'porcelain-like sheen'. The lesions may become ulcerative (35%) and direct trauma to the area should be avoided. These lesions may spontaneously disappear in up to 19% of patients.

### DIFFERENTIAL DIAGNOSIS
Differential diagnosis of this lesion includes granuloma annulare, necrobiotic xanthogranuloma (associated with paraproteinemia), rheumatoid arthritis nodules, sarcoidosis, stasis dermatitis, lichen sclerosus et atrophicus, Hansen's disease, and erythema nodosum.

### DIAGNOSIS
Diagnosis is through history and physical exam as well as familiarity with the lesion.

### MANAGEMENT/TREATMENT
Both medical and surgical treatments of necrobiosis lipodica have been of limited efficacy. In ulcerative or complicated cases, surgery or split-thickness skin grafts have been used. Medical treatments have included topical or intralesion corticosteroids, fibrinolytic agents, nicotinamide, tacrolimus, pentoxifylline, heparin, antiplatelet agents, ticlodipine hydrochloride, tretinoin, cyclosporine, and thalidomide.

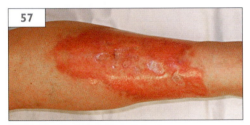

57 Necrobiosis lipoidica diabeticorum. (Courtesy of Drs. Anthony Peterson and David Eilers.)

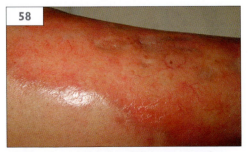

58 Necrobiosis lipoidica diabeticorum with telangiectasia. (Courtesy of Drs. Anthony Peterson and David Eilers.)

# Acanthosis nigricans

### DEFINITION/OVERVIEW
Acanthosis nigricans is a papillomatosis and hyperkeratosis of the skin. The lesions are commonly associated with type 2 diabetes mellitus and hyperinsulinemic states. This lesion may be seen in up to 36% of people with type 2 diabetes. Acanthosis has a higher prevalence in African Americans, Hispanics, and Native Americans when compared with Caucasians.

### ETIOLOGY
Hyperinsulinemic states and obesity are commonly associated with acanthosis nigricans, suggesting that insulin resistance may participate in the genesis of this lesion. The incidence of acanthosis in moderately obese individuals may be as high as 27% and up to 54% in severe obesity.

### PATHOPHYSIOLOGY
Acanthosis nigricans is characterized as a dermal thickening with hyperpigmentation. Acanthosis is thought to arise from insulin stimulation of IGF-1 receptors in keratinocytes leading to epidermal hyperplasia.

### CLINICAL PRESENTATION
The dermal thickening seen in acanthosis appears as dark, velvety areas (**59**). They are commonly distributed to the axilla, neck, back, and periumbilical areas. In diabetic dermopathy, groups of small >5 mm red papules occur on the arms and legs of diabetic individuals. These lesions slowly develop shallow centers and characteristically evolve into hyperpigmented scars.

### DIFFERENTIAL DIAGNOSIS
Rapidly appearing lesions of acanthosis in elderly nonobese patients should prompt the clinician to search for occult malignancy, as there is an association with paraneoplastic syndromes and cancer. Acanthosis nigricans is also associated with polycystic ovarian syndrome, congenital adrenal hyperplasia, Cushing's disease, acromegaly, obesity, and Prader–Willi syndrome.

### DIAGNOSIS
Diagnosis is through history and physical examination as well as familiarity with the lesion. Groups of small >5 mm red papules occur on the arms and legs of diabetics. These lesions slowly develop shallow centers and characteristic hyperpigmentation.

### MANAGEMENT/TREATMENT
Reduction of insulin resistance by weight loss and/or use of metformin or thiazolidinediones may lead to amelioration or even disappearance of acanthosis.

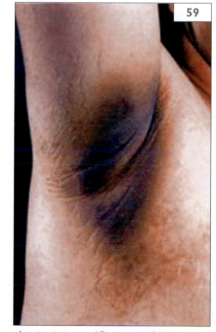

**59** Acanthosis nigricans. (Courtesy of *Mayo Clinic Proceedings*, with permission.)

# Cutaneous infections

### DEFINITION/OVERVIEW
Malignant otitis externa is predominantly seen in elderly patients with glucose intolerance or diabetes mellitus. The most common causative bacterium is *Pseudomonas areuginosa* though it may also, less commonly, be secondary to *Aspergillus*, *Staphylococcus*, *Proteus*, *Klebsiella*, or *Candida*.

Mucormycosis or *Zygomycosis*, is a rare but rapidly growing infection by the class of fungi *Zygomycetes*. They are common in nature, and are aerosolized as spores. In diabetic patients, or patients with metabolic acidosis, the most common and devastating manifestation is rhinocerebral *Mucormycosis*. Almost three-quarters of all cases of rhinocerebral *Mucormycosis* are associated with diabetes.

### PATHOPHYSIOLOGY
*P. aeruginosa* is not a common pathogen of the external ear. It is thought to be introduced by contamination of water. Poor tissue perfusion, secondary to microangiopathy and immuno-compromise increase susceptibility to this infection. The infection may spread to the meninges, brain, or mastoid process. Rhinocerebral *Mucormycosis* most likely begins with the inhalation of spores and the seeding of the nares. The infection begins in the presence of hyperglycemia or metabolic acidosis. The presence of ketone reductase allows the fungi to proliferate in acidic environments and hyperglycemic states.

### CLINICAL PRESENTATION
Patients with malignant otitis media may present with fever and localized ear pain and drainage. Development of meningitis or osteomyelitis may occur. The initial site of infection in diabetic patients is the nasal turbinates. Presentation is consistent with acute sinusitis. Patients may rapidly develop fever, sinus tenderness and pain, purulent discharge, and severe headaches. Spread is to contiguous areas. Common sites include the orbits, palate. and brain. If the etiology of the infection is fungal, there may be marked tissue destruction and angioinvasivion. Nerve palsies, proptosis, facial swelling, and cyanosis of overlying structures may be seen.

### DIFFERENTIAL DIAGNOSIS
Squamous cell carcinoma of the external ear may mimic signs and symptoms of malignant otitis media.

### DIAGNOSIS
Diagnosis of malignant otitis externa is accomplished through history and thorough physical examination. Laboratory values may indicate presence of an infection. The erythrocyte sedimentation rate, although nonspecific, is generally elevated. Biopsy of ear is the only reliable mechanism to differentiate between squamous cell carcinoma and malignant otitis externa. Culture will help determine the causative organism and direct appropriate antimicrobial therapy.

Diagnosis of mucormycosis is via culture. The aggressive nature of the investigation warrants rapid identification. Direct biopsy and staining of necrotic tissue is appropriate. Clinicians should treat patients immediately if suspicion is high. CT scan or MRI should be employed to determine the extent of the disease.

### MANAGEMENT/TREATMENT
Malignant otitis externa may be treated with parenteral combination antibiotics, or single agent fluoroquinolone. Current treatment of rhinocerebral mucormycosis includes aggress-ive and potentially disfiguring debridement. Amphotericin B is the antifungal of choice.

## Diabetic dermopathy

### DEFINITION/OVERVIEW
Diabetic dermopathy is a common finding in patients with long-standing diabetes mellitus and encompasses many types of skin lesions which are not explained by other classifications of skin lesions. It is a diagnosis of exclusion.

### ETIOLOGY
Diabetic dermopathy is associated with long-standing disease. The areas affected suggest a relationship with local trauma.

### DIFFERENTIAL DIAGNOSIS
For dermopathy, cutaneous infections and cancer must be ruled out.

### MANAGEMENT/TREATMENT
There is no specific treatment for diabetic dermopathy.

## Other infections

A more common, though less dramatic, infection is intertrigo (**60**). This is any infectious or noninfectious inflammatory condition of two closely opposed skin surfaces. When infectious in etiology, the most common cause is *Candida*, although it may result from any of a variety of micro-organisms. Treatment consists of treatment of the predisposing factor (e.g. weight loss if possible), topical antifungals, and drying agents.

Tinea infections are also fairly common (**61**). They are caused by the organism *Pityrosporum orbiculare* and are treated by topical antifungal agents.

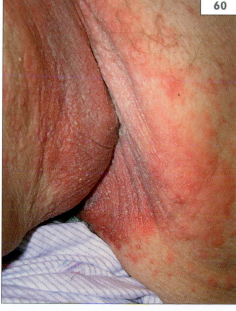

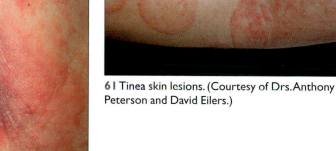

**61** Tinea skin lesions. (Courtesy of Drs. Anthony Peterson and David Eilers.)

**60** Axillary intertrigo. (Courtesy of Dr. Eva Parker.)

# Common drug reactions

### DEFINITION/OVERVIEW

A common finding of drug therapy in diabetes mellitus is localized skin reaction (**62**). Insulin administration may lead to a variety of localized reactions. Hypersensitivity reactions, lipohypertrophy, lipoatrophy, nodule formation, and cellulitus may be seen in patients administered insulin. The use of sufonylureas may lead to the development of a wide variety of skin manifestations. Thiazolidindiones, metformin, and alpha-glucosidase inhibitors have not been associated with significant cutaneous manifestations.

### ETIOLOGY

Please refer to pathophysiology.

### PATHOPHYSIOLOGY

Lipohypertrophy likely results from localized effects of insulin. Insulin in high concentration leads to the inhibition of lipolysis locally. Lipoatrophy is a localized immunologic reaction to the impurities found within the various insulin preparations. Impurities in insulin preparations may cause hypersensitivity reactions locally or systemically. With the use of indwelling catheters associated with insulin pumps, direct skin trauma may lead to hard nodular formations. Additionally, these chronic sites may lead to a port of entry for infections leading to localized cellulitus.

### DIFFERENTIAL DIAGNOSIS

In patients with severe systemic allergic reactions, all medications should be evaluated thoroughly. Vasculitus should be considered in patients with significant skin lesions.

### DIAGNOSIS

Diagnosis of lipohypertrophy, lipoatrophy, and pump-related injury is by history, physical examination, and familiarity with the character of the lesion. Deterioration in glycemic control in patients using the insulin pump may indicate skin problems at the site. Localized cellulitus presents with increasing area of erythema, fevers, and pain.

Sulfonylurea allergic reactions are related temporally to the initiation of therapy and are diagnosed through a thorough history and physical examination. These reactions are typically erythemia multiforme, erythema nodosum, morbilliform rash, or simple puritus. Reactions with the intake of alcohol result in an unpleasant flushing sensation. Second- and third-generation sulfonylureas do not cause this reaction. Jaundice may accompany more severe reactions to sulfonylurea. Photoallergic reactions to ultraviolet B radiation manifest as eruptions on the sun exposed skin: typically hands, face, and neck.

### MANAGEMENT/TREATMENT

Treatment of lipohypertrophy, nodules associated with insulin pumps, and lipoatrophy is simply to vary the site employed for insulin delivery. Patients utilizing insulin pumps should avoid using single sites for greater than 72 hours at a time. Cellulitus should be treated with an appropriate antibiotic regime. Withdrawal of the sulfonylurea is warranted for significant skin changes. In severe reactions, such as the Stevens–Johnson syndrome, hospitalization and supportive care are necessary.

## Bullae

Bullae are rare and tend to appear spontaneously from normal skin (**63**). They are usually on the lower extremities, but sometimes are on the arms, hands, and fingers. They may be intraepidermal or subepidermal. Intraepidermal bullae are sterile and non-hemorrhagic and resolve spontaneously within a few weeks. Subepidermal bullae may be hemorrhagic and may heal with scarring and atrophy. The only therapy is local care to avoid local infection while the lesions resolve spontaneously.

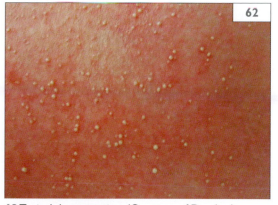

**62** Typical drug eruption. (Courtesy of Drs. Anthony Peterson and David Eilers.)

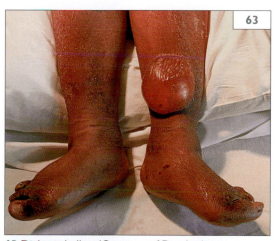

**63** Diabetic bullae. (Courtesy of Drs. Anthony Peterson and David Eilers.)

# The diabetic foot

## DEFINITION/OVERVIEW

The patient with diabetes can have serious foot complications, including ulcers and amputation, largely due to the combined impact of neuropathy and peripheral vascular disease. Diabetic foot ulcers and lower extremity amputations are serious and expensive complications that may affect as many as 15% of people with diabetes during their lifetime. Simple and inexpensive interventions may decrease the amputation rate by up to 85%.

## ETIOLOGY

There are many etiologic and risk factors which can participate in the development of the diabetic foot, especially ulceration. Primarily, diabetic foot disease is a culmination of the combined effects of peripheral neuropathy and peripheral vascular disease. Other factors are associated with increased risk, however. These include increasing duration of diabetes, age, male gender, poor glycemic control, and microvascular and macrovascular diabetic complications. There is a weak association with cigarette smoking (though it should be avoided in any case); alcohol consumption does not have a clear association with foot ulcerations.

## PATHOPHYSIOLOGY

Neuropathy leads to ulceration by several mechanisms. First, there is loss of sensation so that an individual may not recognize the development of ulceration early. Second, the motor component of neuropathy leads to atrophy of the intrinsic muscles of the foot, resulting in a flexion deformity. This results in increased pressure on the metatarsal heads and tips of toe, common places for ulceration (**64**). Third, peripheral sympathetic autonomic neuropathy causes dyshidrosis and dry skin, which can readily crack, allowing for invasion of pathogenic bacteria. Autonomic neuropathy may also be involved with arteriovenous shunting leading to altered skin and bone perfusion. Neuropathy, because of sensory loss, can also lead to the development of Charcot foot and attendant ulceration (**65–67**).

Another pathophysiologic factor is limited joint mobility because of glycosylation of the skin, soft tissue, and joints. This limited joint mobility at the subtalar and first metatarso-phalangeal joint causes higher plantar pressures than in those with normal mobility, and further aggravates the situation caused by the flexion deformity. People with diabetes and neuropathy are more likely to have gait abnormalities making them prone to suffer some kind of injury during ambulation. Calluses may further increase pressure and hemorrhages and early ulcers can form underneath calluses (**68**).

Peripheral vascular disease, highly prevalent in people with diabetes, is an infrequent precipitating event but plays a major role in delayed wound healing and gangrene (**69–71**).

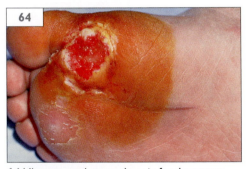

**64** Ulcer secondary to chronic focal pressure callus. (Courtesy of Dr. Ronald Sage.)

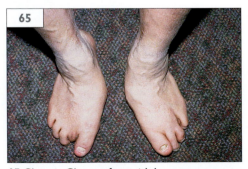

**65** Chronic Charcot feet with hammer toes. (Courtesy of Dr. Ronald Sage.)

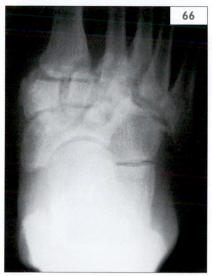

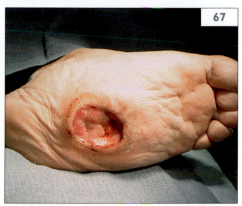

**67** Neuropathic ulcer in Charcot foot. (Courtesy of Dr. Ronald Sage.)

**66** Radiograph of a Charcot foot. (Courtesy of Dr. Laurie Lomasney.)

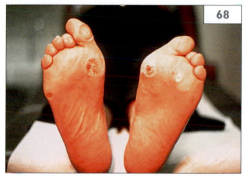

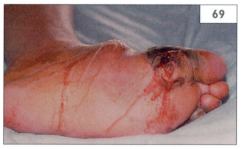

**68** Plantar focal pressure calluses, high risk for ulceration. (Courtesy of Dr. Ronald Sage.)

**69** Extensive limb-threatening ascending infection arising from a first metatarsal ulcer secondary to chronic focal pressure callus. (Courtesy of Dr. Ronald Sage.)

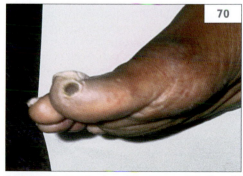

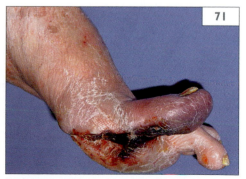

**70** Distal ischemic ulcer. (Courtesy of Dr. Ronald Sage.)

**71** Severe ischemic ulceration, (Courtesy of Dr. Ronald Sage.)

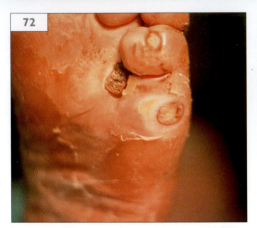

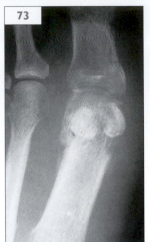

**73** Radiograph showing osteomyelitis. (Courtesy of Dr Laurie Lomasney.)

**72** Ulcer with exposed bone and osteomyelitis. (Courtesy of Dr. Ronald Sage.)

Infection may ultimately lead to osteomyelitis (**72, 73**).

In the context of neuropathy, biomechanical problems, and peripheral vascular disease, a definable precipitating event may start the process of ulceration. This is often poorly fitting footwear.

## CLINICAL PRESENTATION

In its most extreme form, patients with diabetic feet present with foot ulcerations, often infected. Short of this, the presentation is that of peripheral neuropathy, peripheral vascular disease, flexion deformities of the toes, interosseous muscle wasting, dry and cracked skin, and toe nail deformities.

## DIAGNOSIS

A detailed discussion of the many modes of diagnosis of each of the component factors in the development of the diabetic foot (e.g. neuropathy, biomechanical abnormalities, and peripheral neuropathy) is beyond the scope of this discussion. However, in taking the history, attention should be given to classic symptoms of peripheral neuropathy, especially numbness, and classic symptoms of peripheral vascular disease, notably claudication. A previous history of ulceration is also important. The physical examination includes foot inspection to assess for obvious foot deformities, dry skin, cracks in the skin, calluses, and toe nail deformities. Neurologic examination to ascertain whether or not there is sensory loss, and palpation of the pulses should be part of the routine. More specialized procedures such as nerve conduction velocity testing, Doppler, or angiograms may be necessary in some individuals and should be decided on a case-by-case basis.

## MANAGEMENT/TREATMENT

The old axiom that foot inspection prevents amputation remains true. A key part of management is to make sure that the patient and/or a family member looks at the feet daily – top, bottom, and between the toes. Patients should be advised to call their physicians immediately at any sign of infection or anything unusual. The importance of daily self-examination should be reinforced by the physician doing this at every clinic visit. Proper fitting shoes are essential. Patients should be instructed to dry the feet thoroughly after bathing and use skin moisturizers liberally to keep the skin from getting dry and cracking.

The development of peripheral neuropathy can be delayed by good glycemic control, so that is part of the management. Surgical debridement of calluses and good nail care is fundamental. Surgery to correct bony deformities may be indicated. Claudication, a manifestation of peripheral vascular disease, can be managed by a graded exercise program and, in some cases, vascular surgery. Fungal nail infections can be treated with topical and systemic agents.

# Cardiovascular disease in diabetes

## DEFINITION/OVERVIEW
Diabetes mellitus is a well-established independent risk factor for the development and progression of coronary heart disease (CHD), peripheral vascular disease (PVD), and atherosclerotic cerebrovascular disease (CVD). CHD is two- to threefold more common in diabetics than in the general population. Women with diabetes are at a greater risk for the development of CHD than men. The prevalence of symptomatic and silent CHD in this population after age 49 is estimated to be around 30%. The cumulative mortality from CHD is approximately 35% at age 55 in people with type 1 diabetes. Type 2 diabetic patients without known coronary disease had a similar rate of developing a myocardial infarction (MI) (approximately 20%) compared with non-diabetic patients with previous history of myocardial infarction. This was independent of other traditional risk factors. Poor glycemic control is well correlated with the increase in the prevalence of CHD and MI. Carotid arterial disease development and progression is directly correlated with glycemic control. Despite these relationships, no studies have clearly shown the improved glycemic control prevents coronary or carotid disease in type 2 diabetic people. Recent studies have suggested that there might be a delayed macrovascular benefit from periods of antecedent good glycemic control in people with type 1 diabetes. Duration of diabetes mellitus has a significant impact on the development and progression of peripheral arterial disease. Although intensive glycemic control is always advocated, the relationship between glycemic control and peripheral arterial disease treatment has not been well established and no glycemic intervention has been shown to improve PVD.

## ETIOLOGY
The primary defect in cardiovascular disease is the formation and progression of athero-sclerotic plaques, with resultant occlusive or thromboembolic disease. Common risk factors for its development include diabetes mellitus, hypertension, hypercholesterolemia, chronic kidney disease, smoking, obesity, age, and family history.

## PATHOPHYSIOLOGY
Atherosclerosis development is multifactorial. Central to development and progression is endothelial dysfunction. In some patients, there is likely a genetic predisposition to endothelial dysfunction. In other patients, endothelial dysfunction is triggered by hyperglycemia, hypertension, hyperlipidemia, and the products of smoking. At baseline, there appears to be a reduction in the production and release of nitric oxide, a potent vasodilator which has anti-atherosclerotic and antiplatelet properties. Dysfunctional endothelial cells express adhesion molecules which trap circulating monocytes. These are then translocated into the vessel wall itself where they meet a highly oxidative environment. The environment converts the monocytes to macrophages. Low-density lipoprotein (LDL) cholesterol particles also become oxidized within the vessel wall and this process makes them more easily taken up by macrophages. These lipid-laden macro-phages are called foam cells and will eventually rupture, leading to development of the earliest identifiable histologic feature of atherosclerosis, the fatty streak. The oxidized LDL-C particles additionally stimulate tissue macrophages to release proinflammatory cytokines and adhesion molecules, selfperpetuating the inflammatory process.

Hyperglycemia further exacerbates inflammatory cytokine production and oxidative stress. With 60–70% occlusion of a vessel, the patient is likely to experience symptoms. Plaque rupture results in acute syndromes. This phenomenon is typically associated with plaques occluding less than 50% of the vessel lumen. Plaques may additionally undergo remodeling and calcification. Pathology of plaque, plaque rupture, and subsequent ischemic fibrosis is shown in Figures 74–76.

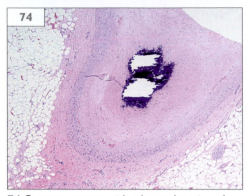

74 Coronary artery with atherosclerosis and calcification. (Courtesy of Dr. Henry Brown.)

## CLINICAL PRESENTATION

Cardiovascular disease diagnosis in the diabetic may present as both a straightforward diagnosis or present with an insidious onset resulting in disastrous consequences. For example, coronary disease can present as sudden death. PVD may initially present with the progression of hair loss in the lower extremities, worsening of neuropathy, an overall cold sensation of the feet, or claudication. Diabetics with pronounced PVD may be predisposed to the development of ulceration and infection. Patients with carotid and cerebrovascular disease present with headache, nausea, syncope, symptoms of stroke, or an early harbinger of severe disease, the transient ischemic attack. Physical examination may reveal carotid bruits and subtle neurologic deficits.

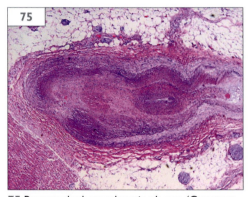

75 Ruptured atherosclerotic plaque. (Courtesy of Dr. Henry Brown.)

## DIAGNOSIS

Physical examination can guide a practitioner in the diagnosis and early treatment of vascular complications of diabetes mellitus. Although powerful imaging and laboratory testing is available, the art of the physical examination remains the cornerstone in diagnosis and stratification of cardiovascular disease. Details of various diagnostic modalities are beyond the scope of this discussion.

## MANAGEMENT/TREATMENT

Acute coronary, peripheral, and cerebral injuries related to arterial insults in diabetic patients should be treated in an emergent fashion under the care of appropriate surgical and acute care physicians. Access to percutaneous coronary angiography and intervention should not be delayed in favor of medical management in patients with non-ST segment elevation MI. Patients should be treated with oxygen, nitrates,

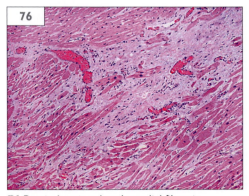

76 Postischemic subendocardial fibrosis. (Courtesy of Dr. Henry Brown.)

antiplatelet agents, beta-blockers, and high-dose statins initially. Patients who have undergone revascularization for CHD should avoid the use of the sulfonylurea glyburide, as in the periprocedure setting this sulfonylurea may reduce the powerful myocardial protection afforded by ischemic preconditioning. Diabetic patients admitted to the hospital or intensive care setting should ideally be managed utilizing glycemic protocols. The use of insulin in hyperglycemic patients should be advocated in this setting, regardless of their previous medical regimen and regardless of whether the patient has an antecedent history of diabetes. Decreased mortality and morbidity have been demonstrated for cardiovascular patients in the surgical and medical intensive care units in many but not all studies with good glycemic control achieved by insulin. A suggested algorithm for the treatment of type 2 diabetes is presented in Figure 77.

Therapy should also be directed at controlling cardiovascular risk factors over the long term. Positive lifestyle changes and control of hypertension, microalbuminuria, and lipids should be instituted aggressively.

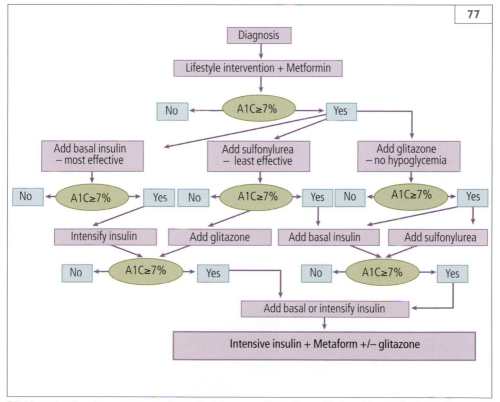

**77** Algorithm for the treatment of type 2 diabetes mellitus. (From Nathan D *et al.* Diabetes Care 2008;**31**:173–5.)

# Secondary causes of diabetes

Although uncommon, it is important not to overlook secondary causes of diabetes associated with physical finds, where treatment could ameliorate the underlying insulin resistance and hyperglycemia. These include acromegaly, excess cortisol states, and glucagonoma.

## Acromegaly
(See also Chapter 4)

### DEFINITION
Acromegaly is almost always caused by a growth hormone (GH)-secreting adenoma of the pituitary gland and is associated with increased morbidity and mortality. GH excess that occurs before fusion of the epiphyseal growth plates in a child or adolescent is called pituitary gigantism; when the excess GH appears in an adult, soft tissue changes are the clinical clues leading to the diagnosis.

### ETIOLOGY
Excess GH stimulates hepatic secretion of IGF-1, which causes most of the clinical manifestations of the disease. The clinical diagnosis is often delayed because of the slow progression of the signs of acromegaly over a period of many years.

### PATHOPHYSIOLOGY
Serum GH concentrations and IGF-1 concentrations are increased in virtually all patients with acromegaly. The increases in serum IGF-1 are often disproportionately greater than are those in GH for two reasons: GH secretion fluctuates more; and GH stimulates the secretion of IGF-1-binding protein-3 (IGFBP-3), the major IGF-1 binding protein in serum. Other rare causes of acromegaly include pituitary somatotroph carcinoma, hypothalamic tumor secreting growth hormone-releasing hormone (GHRH), nonendocrine tumor secreting GHRH, ectopic secretion of GH by a nonendocrine tumor, and excess growth factor activity.

### CLINICAL PRESENTATION
Clinical clues to acromegaly include visual field defects, cranial nerve palsy, acral enlargement including thickness of soft tissue of the hands (**78**) and skin tags, macroglossia, thyromegaly, hepatomegaly, and galactorrhea. These features progress over time (**79**).

### DIAGNOSIS
A normal serum IGF-1 concentration is strong evidence that the patient does not have acromegaly. If the serum IGF-1 concentration

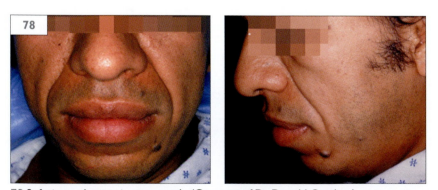

**78** Soft tissue changes in acromegaly. (Courtesy of Dr. Donald Gordon.)

is high (or equivocal), serum GH should be measured after oral glucose administration. It is equally acceptable to proceed immediately to MRI after obtaining an elevated level of IGF-1. If the MRI is normal, then studies to identify a GHRH- or GH-secreting tumor should be undertaken. All patients with acromegaly have increased GH secretion. However, the random serum GH concentration is often in the range of 2–10 ng/mL during much of the day, values that can be found in normal subjects. Unlike normal subjects, the patient's serum GH concentration changes little during the day or night, and in most patients does not change in response to stimuli such as food or exercise. Nevertheless, because of the variations in serum GH that occur in normal subjects and in patients with other disorders, a high value cannot be interpreted without knowing when the blood sample was obtained and something about the patient. To obviate these problems, it is best not to obtain random measurements of serum GH.

The most specific dynamic test for establishing the diagnosis of acromegaly is an oral glucose tolerance test. In normal subjects, serum GH concentrations fall to 1 ng/mL or less within 2 hours after ingestion of 75 g glucose. In contrast, the postglucose values are greater than 2 ng/mL in acromagly.

## TREATMENT/MANAGEMENT

Since acromegaly is associated with increased cardiovascular risk, almost all patients should be treated, even those who are asymptomatic and those in whom the disorder does not seem to be progressing. Selective transsphenoidal surgical resection is the treatment of choice for patients. Surgical resection may be followed up with radiotherapy or medical treatment with analogs of somatostatin (growth hormone-inhibitory hormone) that inhibit GH secretion more effectively than native somatostatin because of their greater potency and longer plasma half-life. These include octreotide and lanreotide. Octreotide is available in short- and long-acting forms; lanreotide is available in long-acting forms.

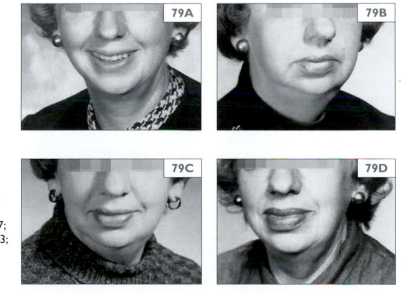

**79** Progression of acromegaly over 11 years. A = 1977; B = 1981; C = 1983; D = 1988. (Courtesy of Dr. Donald Gordon.)

# Excess cortisol states: Cushing's syndrome

(See also Chapters 4 and 5)

## DEFINITION

Excess cortisol can be due to exogenous use (iatrogenic Cushing's syndrome) or due to endogenous causes, which include benign and malignant adrenal tumors, pituitary adrenocorticotrophic hormone (ACTH)-dependent Cushing's syndrome (Cushing's disease), and ectopic ACTH from other malignancies. It is crucial to determine the cause of the excess glucocorticoids so that appropriate treatment can be given.

## ETIOLOGY

Excess cortisol due to exogenous use (iatrogenic Cushing's syndrome) is more common than any other cause, but is seldom reported. Cushing's syndrome may also be caused by a benign adrenal adenoma, often discovered incidentally on radiographic studies. While adrenal nodules are noted in up to 8.7% of adults, they are usually not associated with any clinical adrenal disease. Excess glucocorticoid production, however, is the most common hormone overproduced. A very rare cause of Cushing's syndrome is adrenal carcinoma, which is estimated to be 0.2–2 per million per year. Pituitary ACTH-dependent Cushing's syndrome (Cushing's disease) is due to hypersecretion of pituitary ACTH by the pituitary corticotrophs and is associated with bilateral adrenocortical hyperplasia. It is five to six times more common than Cushing's syndrome caused by benign and malignant adrenal tumors combined, with women three to eight times more likely than men to develop Cushing's disease. Ectopic ACTH syndrome, although often not diagnosed, can cause Cushing's syndrome; about 1% of patients with small-cell lung cancer have ectopic ACTH syndrome and small-cell lung carcinoma causes half of all cases of the syndrome.

## PATHOPHYSIOLOGY

ACTH-dependent Cushing's syndrome is due to hypersecretion of pituitary ACTH by the corticotrophs and is associated with bilateral adrenocortical hyperplasia. There is loss of synchrony between ACTH and cortisol secretion, with hypersecretion of cortisol and the loss of normal circadian rhythm. Morning plasma ACTH and serum cortisol concentrations may be normal, but late-evening concentrations are high. Salivary cortisol concentrations reflect those of serum free cortisol. The increased cortisol secretion is reflected by increased urinary excretion of cortisol. The pituitary adenoma cells function at a higher than normal set point for cortisol feedback inhibition, and this characteristic is clinically important because it permits the use of dexamethasone suppression to distinguish between pituitary and ectopic ACTH secretion; the latter is usually very resistant to glucocorticoid negative feedback. Almost all patients with Cushing's disease have a pituitary adenoma, although the tumor is often not demonstrable by imaging; the remainder have corticotroph hyperplasia. The tumors are usually microadenomas; only about 5% are macroadenomas. Patients with macroadenomas are more likely to have high plasma ACTH concentrations than are those with microadenomas, and the concentrations are less likely to fall with high doses of dexamethasone. Patients with ectopic ACTH secretion will have persistent cortisol elevation, even with high-dose dexamethasone testing. Adrenal adenomas, which are almost always benign, can also oversecrete cortisol, but the concomitant ACTH level will be suppressed.

## CLINICAL PRESENTATION

Clinical clues to the diagnosis of Cushing's disease are underlying centripetal obesity, facial plethora, impaired glucose tolerance or type 2 diabetes, proximal muscle weakness, hypertension, easy bruising, hirsutism, depression, oligomenorrhea, acne, abdominal striae, and edema (**80**).

## DIAGNOSIS

The diagnosis of Cushing's disease involves suspicion on the basis of the patient's symptoms and signs, documenting the presence of hypercortisolemia, and determining its cause.

## MANAGEMENT/TREATMENT

If a patient is taking exogenous steroids, discontinuation is recommended if this is possible. If a cortisol-producing adrenal adenoma is found, surgical removal should be curative. If a pituitary adenoma is responsible

(Cushing's disease), then neurosurgical intervention is the procedure of choice often followed by radiation therapy. If ectopic ACTH secretion is determined to be the source, treatment of the underlying malignancy is needed.

# Glucagonoma
(See also Chapter 8)

## DEFINITION
Glucagonomas are rare islet cell tumors of the pancreas which oversecrete glucagon. The systemic manifestations make it unique among islet cell tumors and provide visible clues that make early diagnosis possible.

## ETIOLOGY
Nearly all reported cases of the glucagonoma syndrome have been associated with tumors originating in the alpha cells of the pancreas. These tumors demonstrate the typical characteristics of islet cell tumors: they are usually encapsulated, firm nodules, varying in size from 2 cm up to 25 cm, and occur most often in the tail of the pancreas.

## PATHOPHYSIOLOGY
Glucagonomas consist of cords and nests of well-differentiated islet cells. Characteristic alpha cell granules may be seen on electron microscopy. Despite their benign histologic appearance, most pancreatic glucagonomas are malignant, as defined by their propensity for metastasis which is usually present at the time of diagnosis.

## CLINICAL PRESENTATION
Patients typically present in their fifth decade, with an even distribution between males and females. The clinical syndrome classically associated with glucagonoma includes necrolytic migratory erythema (**81**), cheilitis, diabetes mellitus, anemia, weight loss, venous thrombosis, and neuropsychiatric symptoms. Weight loss and necrolytic migratory erythema are the most prevalent symptoms, occurring in approximately 65–70% of patients by the time of diagnosis. Necrolytic migratory characteristically begins as erythematous papules or plaques involving the face, perineum, and extremities. Over the next 7–14 days, the lesions enlarge and coalesce. Central clearing then occurs, leaving bronze-colored, indurated

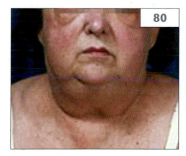

80 Clinical features of Cushing's disease. (Courtesy of Dr. Donald Gordon.)

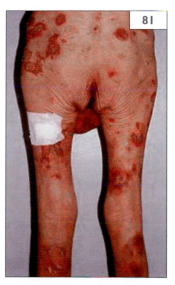

81 Skin manifestations of glucogonoma syndrome. (Courtesy of Donald Gordon.)

lesions. The rash may occasionally appear prior to the onset of systemic symptoms, but most patients with rash usually have weight loss, diarrhea, sore mouth, weakness, mental status changes, or diabetes mellitus. Venous thrombosis occurs in up to 30% of patients with glucagonoma; this association with thromboembolism appears to be unique among endocrine tumors. Neurologic symptoms associated with glucagonoma may include ataxia, dementia, optic atrophy, and proximal muscle weakness. The prevalence of metastatic disease at the time of diagnosis varies from 50–100%, with the most common sitse of metastasis being the liver, followed by regional lymph nodes, bone, adrenal gland, kidney, and lung. Rarely, glucagonoma may be associated with MEN1; such patients typically have a family history of pituitary, pancreatic islet cell, or parathyroid tumors.

### DIAGNOSIS
The characteristic skin lesion of the glucagonoma syndrome is often the clue which leads to the correct diagnosis, and the presence of necrolytic migratory erythema should prompt further work-up. A serum glucagon level should be obtained. It is important to recognize, however, that conditions other than glucagonoma can induce 'physiologic' elevations in the serum glucagon concentration. These include hypoglycemia, fasting, trauma, sepsis, acute pancreatitis, abdominal surgery, Cushing's syndrome, and renal and hepatic failure. However, these conditions are associated with only moderate elevations of glucagon, usually less than 500 pg/mL (upper limit of normal <100 pg/mL), while a glucagonoma is associated with markedly elevated glucagon concentrations. This should be followed up with an abdominal CT. Since the tumor is usually large by the time of diagnosis, it is localizable by CT in the majority of cases. Endoscopic ultrasonography can detect pancreatic tumors as small as 2–3 mm, provides accurate information on the local extent of disease, and is the modality of choice for detecting and biopsy of islet cell tumors too small for CT visualization. Finally, somatostatin receptor scintigraphy using radiolabeled octreotide is very sensitive for glucagonomas; however, since these tumors are usually large by the time of diagnosis, this is rarely required for diagnosis.

### MANAGEMENT/TREATMENT
For the minority of cases in which the tumor remains localized at the time of diagnosis, resection of the primary pancreatic tumor is indicated since it offers the chance of complete cure. Whether a simple enucleation, focal pancreatic resection, or Whipple procedure is performed is dictated by the site and extent of the tumor. Because patients with glucagonoma syndrome suffer from a prolonged catabolic state, nutritional support of some kind is an integral component of therapy. Treatment for metastatic disease includes somatostatin analogs such as octreotide and lanreotide. Finally, interferon improves symptoms of hormonal hypersecretion in 40–50% of patients with pancreatic islet cell.

## Therapeutic options for type 2 diabetes

Many options are available to clinicians caring for individuals with diabetes, and it is beyond the scope of this Atlas to review them. A very helpful algorithm is included with the recommendations of the American Diabetes Association for managing out-patient diabetes (77).

# Metabolic bone disorders

Cyprian Gardine

Pauline M Camacho

**Osteoporosis**

**Primary hyperparathyroidism**

**Hypoparathyroidism and
    pseudohypoparathyroidism**

**Paget's disease**

**Osteomalacia**

**Sclerotic bone disorders**

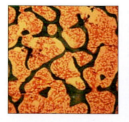
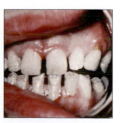
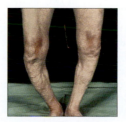
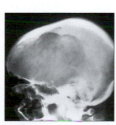

# Osteoporosis

## DEFINITION/OVERVIEW

Osteoporosis is a chronic progressive disease characterized by low bone density, micro-architectural bone deterioration, and decreased bone strength leading to increased bone fragility and increased fracture risk. In 1994 the World Health Organization (WHO) published criteria for the diagnosis of osteoporosis based upon bone mineral density (BMD). Normal BMD is defined as a BMD value within 1 standard deviation of the young adult female reference mean and is designated as a T-score ≥−1. The young adult female reference mean is calculated from the mean BMD of healthy females aged 20–29 of a single ethnicity. Low bone mass (osteopenia) is defined as a BMD that is between 1 and 2.5 standard deviations below the young adult mean and is designated as a T-score <−1 and >−2.5. Osteoporosis is defined as a BMD 2.5 standard deviations or more below the young adult mean designated as a T-score <−2.5. Lastly, severe osteoporosis is defined as a BMD 2.5 standard deviations or more below the young adult mean in the presence of one or more fragility fractures. In current clinical practice, the diagnosis of osteoporosis is based either upon the WHO criteria described above or the presence of fragility fractures. These types of fractures occur with low-impact trauma, such as falling from a standing position.

## ETIOLOGY

Osteoporosis is the most common bone disease in humans. Approximately 33.6 million Americans have osteopenia or low bone mass and 10 million have osteoporosis, of whom 80% are females and 20% are males. The disease affects people of all ethnicities to varying degrees. Non-Hispanic white and Asian people have the greatest incidence of osteoporosis followed by Hispanics and then non-Hispanic blacks. Osteoporosis is responsible for more than 1.5 million fractures annually. One in two women and one in four men over the age of 50 will have an osteoporosis-related fracture during their lifetime. The national health care costs for osteoporosis exceed $20 billion annually. Osteoporosis can be classified as either primary or secondary. Primary osteoporosis is bone loss associated with the aging process. Bone loss in secondary osteoporosis has multiple etiologies (*Table 6*).

## PATHOPHYSIOLOGY

Bone is dynamic. It is constantly undergoing formation and breakdown under the coordinated actions of osteoblasts and osteoclasts. Approximately 5–10% of the adult skeleton is replaced annually through a process called remodeling. Remodeling occurs at focal sites termed 'bone remodeling units'. At these sites, osteoclasts and osteoblasts function in concert to replace old bone with new bone (**82**).

The process begins with bone resorption by osteoclasts. Mononuclear cells proceed to line the resorption lacunae and deposit a cement line. Osteoprogenitor cells replace the mononuclear cells in the bone remodeling unit. These cells differentiate into osteoblasts and begin to lay down the organic matrix. This is then followed by the deposition of minerals. Osteoporosis occurs due to aberrancy in bone remodeling in that there is an increase in osteoclast activity with a concomitant decrease in osteoblast activity. There is also an increase in the total number of bone remodeling units. Therefore, bone resorption is occurring at more sites than usual and in the presence of impaired bone formation. The actions occurring at the bone remodeling unit are under the influence of multiple factors such as estrogen, testosterone, and cytokines.

## CLINICAL PRESENTATION

Osteoporosis is often called a 'silent disease' because bone loss occurs without symptoms. It usually presents as either a fragility fracture or is discovered on radiographic imaging. There are several risk factors associated with osteoporosis including: advanced age, being female, an estrogen deficient state, family history of osteoporosis, history of fracture after age 50, current low bone mass, cigarette smoking, being thin, anorexia nervosa, low calcium intake, vitamin D deficiency, low testosterone, inactive lifestyle, excessive use of alcohol, being Caucasian or Asian, chronic illness, and various medications. On examination the patient may have severe back pain, loss of height, or spinal deformities, such as kyphosis or stooped posture. Other findings may point toward osteoporosis risk factors leading to further diagnostic work-up for osteoporosis.

**Table 6  Secondary causes of osteoporosis**

| Endocrine | Rheumatologic | Drugs | Gastro-intestinal | Hematologic diseases | Other |
|---|---|---|---|---|---|
| Hyperthyroidism | Rheumatoid arthritis | Glucocorticoids | Celiac sprue | Multiple myeloma | Renal insufficiency |
| Primary hyperparathyroidism | SLE | Anticonvulsants | IBD | Mastocytosis | End-organ failure |
| Cushing's syndrome | | | Other malabsorptive syndromes | | Organ transplantation |
| Hypogonadism | | Lithium | Whipples' procedure | | Malnutrition |
| Vitamin D deficiency Calcium deficiency | | Cytotoxic drugs | Gastric by-pass surgery | | Alcoholism |
| | | Heparin | | | HIV |
| | | Aromatase inhibitors | | | COPD |
| | | Gonadotropin releasing hormone agonist | | | Prolonged nonweight bearing states |
| | | Immuno-suppressants | | | |

COPD: chronic obstructive pulmonary disease;  HIV: human immunodeficiency virus;  IBD: inflammatory bowel disease;  SLE: systemic lupus erythematosus.

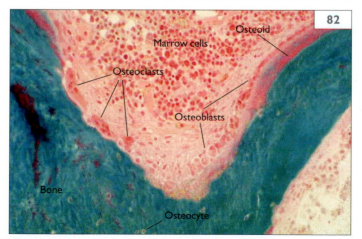

**82** Photomicrograph of bone consisting of a bone remodeling unit comprised of osteoclasts and osteoblasts. (Courtesy of Dr. Susan Ott, with permission, http://courses.washington.edu/bonephys/ophome.html.)

Osteoporosis is associated with increased bone fragility and increased fracture risk. Hip fractures are the most devastating complication of osteoporosis, and 90% of hip fractures occur in patients over the age of 50. One out of every six Caucasian women will have a hip fracture during their lifetime. There is a 10–20% excess mortality in the first year after a hip fracture. The diagnosis, treatment, and prevention of osteoporosis result in a considerable decrease in the incidence of fractures and, therefore, a decrease in mortality and morbidity.

## DIFFERENTIAL DIAGNOSIS

The differential diagnosis includes osteomalacia, malignancy, and the myriad of secondary causes of osteoporosis.

## DIAGNOSIS

Dual energy X-ray absorptiometry (DXA) scan of the lumbar spine and femoral neck is the most common way to diagnose osteoporosis. Other imaging modalities include quantitative ultrasound, quantitative CT, and radiography. Compared to DXA scanning, quantitative ultrasound is unable to provide diagnostic criteria, quantitative CT is more expensive and involves greater radiation exposure, and radiography is less sensitive. DXA provides information regarding bone mineral density and using reference means can provide both T-scores and Z-scores. Z-scores compare the individual's bone density with age-matched controls. In postmenopausal women and in men over age 50, T-scores have the greatest validity. In premenopausal women and men under age 50, Z-scores have the most validity. The reference mean for Z-scores should be age and ethnicity appropriate, particularly in children.

Histopathologic findings in osteoporosis include cortical thinning, increased cortical porosity, and thin trabeculae (**83**), and bone densitometry reveals decreased bone mineral density (**84, 85**). Radiography may reveal compression fractures of the spine (**86**).

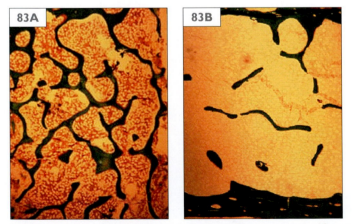

**83** Bone biopsies. **A**: Normal trabecular bone; **B**: osteoporosis. (Courtesy of Dr. Susan Ott, with permission, http://courses.washington.edu/bonephys/ophome.html.)

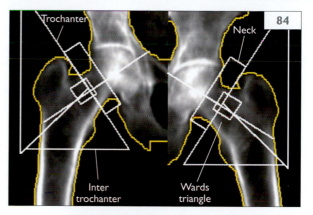

**84** Dual energy X-ray absorptiometry of the left and right hip from a patient with severe osteoporosis. The regions are labeled. The total hip is the sum of the regions.

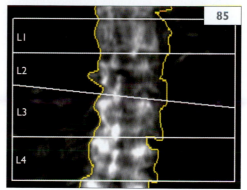

**85** Dual energy X-ray absorptiometry of the lumbar spine. The yellow and white lines are added to the image to guide the scanner software in calculating the bone density.

### MANAGEMENT/TREATMENT

The treatment and prevention of osteoporosis begins with nonpharmacologic therapies. Daily calcium and vitamin D intake should be optimized. In premenopausal women the daily elemental calcium intake should be 1000 mg/d. At menopause that should be increased to 1200–1500 mg/d. Similarly, men should optimize their elemental calcium intake to 1000 mg/d until age 65 and then increase it to 1500 mg/d. The daily intake of vitamin D for adults should be 400–600 IU. In patients at risk of vitamin D deficiency, such as the elderly and chronically ill, the daily intake of vitamin D should be 800 IU.

Exercise is recommended in the treatment and prevention of osteoporosis. Weight bearing exercise helps to maintain or increase bone mass. Regular exercise improves strength and coordination which reduces the risk of falls. Fall prevention is important in the treatment and prevention of osteoporosis. Interventions that reduce the risk of falls are essential. Risk factors for falls include visual impairment, poor balance

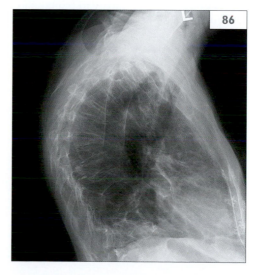

**86** Lateral radiograph of a patient with severe osteoporosis revealing kyphosis secondary to multiple vertebral fractures.

or gait, neuromuscular and musculoskeletal disabilities, muscle weakness, postural hypotension, medications, cognitive impairment, and environmental hazards. Cessation of habits such as cigarette smoking and excessive alcohol consumption are suggested in the treatment and prevention of osteoporosis.

Pharmacologic intervention is recommended for patients with a BMD T-score below –2.0, patients with a BMD T-score below –1.5 if additional osteoporosis risk factors are present, and any patient with a previous vertebral or hip fracture. The medications employed in the treatment of osteoporosis include oral bisphosphonates, raloxifene, estrogen/progesterone replacement therapy, nasal calcitonin, and teriparatide. The primary goal in the treatment of osteoporosis is to reduce the incidence of fractures. A secondary goal is to maintain and if possible normalize the BMD.

Bisphosphonates block bone resorption by inhibiting the activity of osteoclasts. Currently they are the most potent antiresorptive agents available for the treatment and prevention of osteoporosis. Strong clinical trial evidence supports the use of alendronate, risedronate, ibandronate, and zoledronic acid for preventing fractures in women with postmenopausal osteoporosis or osteopenia and in men with osteoporosis. These agents have been shown to reduce vertebral fractures by 50–70% and hip fractures by 40% in postmenopausal women. Oral bisphosphonates are contraindicated in patients with esophageal irritation or stricture, hypocalcemia, hypersensitivity to bisphosphonates, or renal insufficiency (creatinine clearance <30 mL/min). Rarely patients may develop osteonecrosis of the jaw. The 10-year efficacy and safety data have been published for alendronate therapy and 7-year data for risedronate.

Raloxifene is a selective estrogen receptor modulator that is approved for both the treatment and the prevention of postmenopausal osteoporosis. In clinical studies raloxifene has been shown to decrease vertebral fractures by about 50%. However, no evidence is currently available for raloxifene that assesses hip fracture reduction.

The use of estrogen/progesterone replacement therapy remains controversial in the treatment of osteoporosis. Estrogen alone or in combination with progesterone decreases bone turnover, bone loss, and fractures. Due to the risks associated with estrogen/progesterone therapy, it is recommended that other proven therapies such as bisphosphonates are used in the treatment and prevention of osteoporosis. If estrogen/progesterone therapy is desired, the lowest possible dose over the shortest possible time is suggested.

Calcitonin inhibits bone resorption by osteoclasts. It is usually administered as a nasal spray. In clinical studies nasal calcitonin has been shown to prevent bone loss and vertebral fractures. However, it has not been shown to reduce nonvertebral or hip fractures. Because of its modest effect on osteoporosis treatment, this drug is mostly used as an alternative agent.

Teriparatide is a recombinant human parathyroid hormone (PTH) analog. It has been shown to be a potent bone anabolic agent that increases bone turnover. Studies show that teriparatide increases bone density, and reduces vertebral fractures by 65% and nonvertebral fractures by 53%. Its use is recommended in postmenopausal women with severe bone loss who are at high risk for fracture, as well as for the treatment of hypogonadal or primary osteoporosis in men at high risk for fracture. Teriparatide should not be used in patients with a history of bone malignancy, Paget's disease of bone, unexplained hypercalcemia, skeletal radiation exposure, or those younger than 18 years.

Combination therapy with two antiresorptive agents shows some BMD benefit but no fracture reduction data. There is evidence to support sequential use of anabolic followed by antiresorptive therapy, and conflicting evidence on combination therapy.

# Primary hyperparathyroidism

## DEFINITION/OVERVIEW
Hyperparathyroidism is a disease defined by the overproduction of PTH. It can be classified as primary, secondary, or tertiary. Primary hyperparathyroidism (PHP) is characterized by hypercalcemia due to the autonomous overproduction of PTH, either as a result of parathyroid cell proliferation or impaired calcium sensing ability. Secondary hyperparathyroidism is the overproduction of PTH due to hypocalcemia and vitamin D deficiency. Tertiary hyperparathyroidism is the development of autonomous parathyroid function manifested as hypercalcemia and elevated PTH in patients with long-standing secondary hyperparathyroidism.

## ETIOLOGY
PHP is present in about 1% of the adult population. The incidence of the disease increases to 2% or higher after age 55 years. PHP is two to three times more common in women than in men. Approximately 80–85% of cases of PHP are caused by a single parathyroid adenoma. The remainder are due to multiple gland hyperplasia affecting all parathyroid glands (10% of cases), double adenomas (4% of cases), and parathyroid carcinoma (1% of cases). PHP is most commonly due to a sporadic parathyroid adenoma, but may be inherited in endocrine syndromes such as MEN type 1, MEN type 2A, familial hyperparathyroidism, and hyperparathyroidism jaw tumor syndrome. Associated risk factors include neck irradiation and treatment with lithium.

## PATHOPHYSIOLOGY
Solitary parathyroid adenomas are monoclonal or oligoclonal tumors most frequently arising from somatic or germline mutations in parathyroid precursor cells. Several genes that develop mutations in PHP have been identified. The MEN type 1 gene is a tumor suppressor gene and the gene known to most frequently have somatic mutations in both copies in parathyroid adenomas. Activating mutations of the cyclin D1 gene resulting in the overexpression of the protein cyclin D1 have been identified in parathyroid adenomas.

Activating mutations in the RET proto-oncogene have also been identified in parathyroid adenomas. Of note, although the calcium sensing receptor and the vitamin D receptor mediate inhibition of the parathyroid gland, no mutations of these genes have been isolated in parathyroid adenomas.

In secondary hyperparathyroidism the elevated PTH is a physiologic response to hypocalcemia. Hypocalcemia can be due to chronic renal disease. In chronic renal disease hyperphosphatemia impairs the ability of the kidneys to reabsorb calcium, resulting in hypercalciuria and hypocalcemia. Additionally, there is impaired conversion of 25-hydroxy vitamin to 1,25-dihydroxy vitamin D in the diseased kidney, the active form of vitamin D. It is a calcemic agent regulating calcium and phosphate transport as well as a cell differentiating agent important for a number of cell types including the osteoclast, enterocyte, and keratinocyte. Ultimately, deficiency of 1,25-dihydroxy vitamin D results in hypocalcemia which is a stimulus to the parathyroid cells to produce PTH.

Hypocalcemia can also be due to vitamin D deficiency. Vitamin D, although termed a vitamin, is in fact better described as a prohormone. The term vitamin D includes a large group of closely related seco steroids. Cholecalciferol is the form of vitamin D obtained when radiant energy from the sun strikes the skin and converts 7-dehydrocholesterol into vitamin $D_3$. Vitamin D deficiency can occur when there is decreased exposure to the sun, decreased dietary intake of foods containing vitamin D, or decreased absorption of vitamin D from the diet due to malabsorption syndromes such as celiac sprue. Whatever the cause for the low vitamin D, as described above, it is essential for calcium homeostasis.

## CLINICAL PRESENTATION
In the past, the classic clinical presentation of PHP consisted of 'stones, moans, and groans', i.e. nephrolithiasis, osteoporosis, fractures, gout, peptic ulcer disease, pancreatitis, fatigue, anxiety, depression, and cognitive dysfunction.

Other manifestations of PHP include muscle weakness, fatigue, renal insufficiency, hypomagnesemia, hypophosphatemia, hypertension, left ventricular hypertrophy, valvular calcifications, vascular stiffness, chondrocalcinosis, pseudogout, normochromic and normocytic anemia, and band keratopathy (**87**). Essentially clinical manifestations of PHP are all secondary to the induced hypercalcemia, hypercalciuria, and increased bone turnover. With the inclusion of the total calcium on the basic metabolic panel, most patients are diagnosed early in the course of PHP secondary to hypercalcemia. Consequently, patients are often asymptomatic or have subtle neurobehavioral symptoms such as fatigue and weakness.

As most patients with PHP are asymptomatic, the physical examination often fails to lead to a definitive diagnosis. Careful examination may reveal proximal muscle weakness or illicit nonspecific symptoms, such as depression, lethargy, and vague aches and pains. Diagnosis is usually dependent upon biochemical tests.

**DIFFERENTIAL DIAGNOSIS**

The differential diagnosis of hypercalcemia mainly includes cancer, milk-alkali syndrome, granulomatous disease, hyperthyroidism, thiazide diuretics, lithium, and familial hypocalciuric hypercalcemia. A normal or elevated PTH excludes malignancy, calcium and vitamin D toxicity and granulomatous diseases.

**DIAGNOSIS**

The diagnosis of PHP requires determination of serum total or ionized calcium and intact PTH. The 24-hour urinary calcium should be obtained to rule out familial hypocalciuric hypercalcemia. A calcium to creatinine clearance ratio below 0.01 differentiates patients with familial hypocalciuric hypercalcemia from those with PHP. Associated laboratory abnormalities include decreased serum phosphate levels, high normal or increased serum chloride levels, elevated levels of blood urea nitrogen, elevated levels of creatinine, and elevated levels of bone-specific alkaline phosphatase. Patients with PHP should have a bone densitometry scan performed to ascertain the presence or absence of osteopenia or osteoporosis. Parathyroid imaging has no role in the diagnosis of PHP, but ultrasonography or sestamibi scanning of the parathyroid glands should be used for operative planning. Imaging can aid in localizing the parathyroid adenoma(s) to particular parathyroid glands (**88**).

Histology of the parathyroid gland in hyperparathyroidism can distinguish between malignancy and hypercellular causes such as adenoma and hyperplasia. Histologically, normal parathyroid tissue shows a cell to fat ratio of 1:1. Hypercellular parathyroid tissue is typified by the loss of the normal amount of fat. The classic radiographic findings in PHP include nephrolithiasis (**89**), subperiosteal resorption (**90**), thinning of the distal third of the clavicle (**91**), and osteitis fibrosa cystica (**92**).

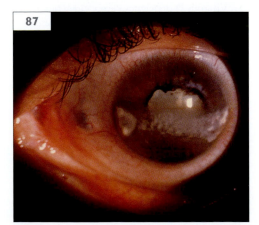

**87** Band keratopathy in a patient with hyperparathyroidism. The name is derived from the distinctive appearance of calcium deposition in a band across the central cornea. (Courtesy of Dr. Glen Sizemore.)

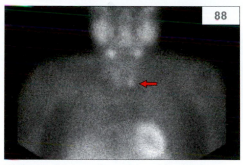

88 Sestamibi scan of a patient with a left lower parathyroid adenoma (arrow). The patient's salivary glands (parotid, submandibular, and sublingual) represent the bright areas around the jaw.

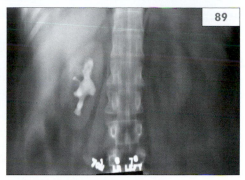

89 Abdominal radiograph showing nephrolithiasis in the right renal medulla in a patient with hyperparathyroidism. (Courtesy of Dr. Glen Sizemore.)

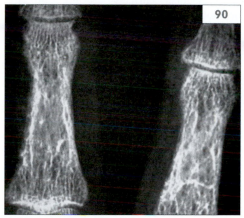

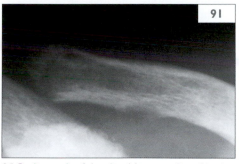

91 Radiograph of the shoulder revealing thinning of the distal third of the clavicle in a patient with hyperparathyroidism. (Courtesy of Dr. Glen Sizemore.)

90 Radiograph of the hands revealing subperosteal bone resorption of the digits in a patient with hyperparathyroidism. (Courtesy of Dr. Glen Sizemore.)

92 A photomicrograph of a bone biopsy revealing osteitis fibrosis. This occurs in patients with hyperpara-thyroidism from increased osteoclastic resorption of calcified bone with replacement by fibrous tissue resulting in softened and deformed bone that may develop cysts. Region C is magnified and made into another image on the following website: Dr. Susan Ott, with permission, http://courses.washington.edu/bonephys/ophome.html.

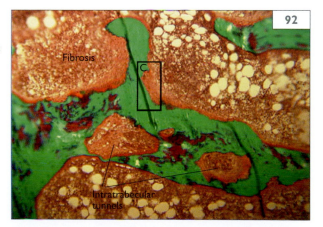

## MANAGEMENT/TREATMENT

Surgery is the first-line treatment for PHP in patients who are symptomatic. The best management for asymptomatic patients with PHP is more controversial. The 2009 Guidelines for the Management of Asymptomatic Primary Hyperparathyroidism (Third International Workshop) recommends surgery for patients who fulfill the following criteria:

1) Serum calcium >1.0 mg/dl (0.25 mmol/l) upper limit of normal.
2) Creatinine clearance <60 mg/min.
3) T score <−2.5 at any site and/or previous fracture fragility.
4) Age <50 years.

Preoperative localization is optional in patients without previous neck surgery. Technetium 99m sestamibi scan and thyroid ultrasound have sensitivities in the range of 60–70%. Intraoperative PTH monitoring guides surgeons while doing minimally invasive parathyroid surgeries.

Medical management is used for those patients who do not meet surgical criteria or who refuse surgery. Patients are instructed to maintain adequate hydration, avoid thiazide diuretics, and limit their dietary intake of calcium to less than 1000 mg/day. Several medications have been shown to be of benefit in treating PHP. Bisphosphonates inhibit bone resorption, but persistent lowering of serum calcium has not been shown. Estrogen/ progesterone has been shown to increase bone density in postmenopausal women with PHP and some studies indicate that it can decrease serum calcium levels. However, the risks of hormone therapy must be weighed against the benefits for the treatment of PHP. Estrogen/ progesterone are not first-line agents. Calcium sensing receptor agonists act directly on parathyroid cells by way of the calcium sensing receptor in order to inhibit the secretion of PTH. These calcimimetic agents may prove beneficial in the treatment of PHP. Currently they are approved for the treatment of secondary hyperparathyroidism and parathyroid cancer.

In secondary hyperparathyroidism, the goal is to reduce PTH levels to appropriate goals depending on kidney function. In vitamin D deficiency, treatment with ergocalciferol or cholecalciferol usually results in the normalization of the vitamin D level and the concomitant normalization of the calcium and PTH. In renal disease the administration of calcium salts and 1,25-dihydroxy vitamin $D_3$ or calcitriol usually results in the normalization of the serum calcium level. The calcium salts increase the calcium available for absorption and also chelate the phosphate in the intestines. Calcitriol acts at the kidneys, intestines, and bone to decrease calcium renal loss, increase calcium absorption, and increase bone mobilization. As the calcium normalizes, the PTH level also normalizes. Calcimimetic agents as described above are currently approved for treatment of secondary hyperparathyroidism. In some case of severe secondary hyperparathyroidism and tertiary hyperparathyroidism in renal failure, parathyroidectomy may be required.

# Hypoparathyroidism and pseudohypoparathyroidism

## DEFINITION/OVERVIEW

Hypoparathyroidism is defined as low serum calcium and low or inappropriately normal PTH. Pseudohypoparathyroidism is defined as low serum calcium, elevated serum phosphate, and elevated serum PTH.

## ETIOLOGY

The most common cause of hypoparathyroidism is injury to or removal of the parathyroid glands during neck surgery. It most frequently occurs after near total or total thyroidectomy for thyroid carcinoma, occurring in 1–2% of patients. Postsurgical hypoparathyroidism may be transient, permanent, or even intermittent. Other causes of hypoparathyroidism can be categorized as developmental defects in the parathyroid gland, defects in the PTH molecule, defective regulation of PTH secretion, autoimmune hypoparathyroidism, defects in the type 1 PTH receptor, and defects of the stimulatory guanine nucleotide-binding protein.

## PATHOPHYSIOLOGY

DiGeorge syndrome is a congenital defect resulting in the agenesis of the parathyroid glands. The manifestations of this syndrome include conotruncal cardiac defects, facial malformations, learning disability, and incomplete development in the brachial arches, resulting in varying degrees of parathyroid and thymic hypoplasia. DiGeorge syndrome has been shown to be associated with rearrangements and microdeletions affecting an unknown gene or genes on the long arm of chromosome 22.

Defects in the PTH molecule have been shown to result in hypoparathyroidism. A few cases of familial hypoparathyroidism have been described in which the cause was a mutation in the gene for PTH. The mutation resulted in the synthesis of a defective PTH molecule and undetectable amounts of PTH in serum.

Hypoparathyroidism can arise from defective regulation of PTH secretion. Autosomal dominant hypercalciuric hypocalcemia is caused by activating mutations of the parathyroid and renal calcium sensing receptor that result in hypocalcemia and hypercalciuria. The mutations cause excessive calcium-induced inhibition of PTH secretion. The hypocalcemia is usually mild and asymptomatic.

Hypoparathyroidism can occur as a consequence of autoimmunity. Autoimmune polyglandular syndrome type 1 consists of hypoparathyroidism, candidiasis, adrenal insufficiency, and primary hypogonadism, as well as the less common features of malabsorption, gastrointestinal disorders, hypothyroidism, and diabetes. The syndrome is inherited as an autosomal recessive trait and is caused by mutations in an autoimmune regulator gene with a known sequence but an unknown function.

Defects in the type 1 PTH receptor can result in low PTH levels. Jansen's chondrodystrophy is caused by activating mutations of the type 1 PTH receptor. It is characterized by short limbs, mild hypercalcemia, and low serum PTH concentrations. Due to the fact that the serum calcium level is mildly elevated, it does not fulfill the definition of hypoparathyroidism.

Pseudohypoparathyroidism occurs due to PTH resistance as a consequence of defects in the PTH receptor-associated stimulatory guanine nucleotide-binding protein. It is characterized by hypocalcemia and hyperphosphatemia due to resistance to PTH. There are several forms of pseudohypoparathyroidism. Patients with type 1a have hypocalcemia, hyperphosphatemia, elevated PTH levels, hormone resistance to thyrotropin and gonadotropins, and display characteristic physical features that are collectively termed Albright's hereditary osteodystrophy (AHD).

Typically, patients have short stature, round facies, brachydactyly (**93, 94**), obesity, and ectopic soft tissue or dermal ossification(s). In the calvaria, this may manifest as hyperostosis frontalis interna. Intracranial calcification(s) (**95**), cataracts, band keratopathy, subcutaneous calcifications, and dental hypoplasia (**96**) are also common but are likely the consequences of long-standing hypocalcemia. Type 1b patients present predominantly with renal PTH resistance and lack any features of AHO.

Patients with type 1c present with both Albright's hereditary osteodystrophy and PTH resistance but have normal stimulatory guanine nucleotide-binding protein function. Type 2 patients present with a normal urinary cyclic adenosine monophosphate (cAMP) response to PTH but lack a phosphaturic response. Furthermore, they lack any signs of AHO or resistance to other hormones. Lastly, patients with type 2 disease do not display a familial origin.

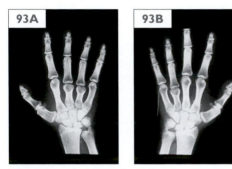

93 Radiographs of a patient's hands.
**A**: Brachydactyly of the third and fourth digits;
**B**: brachydactyly of the fourth digit. (Courtesy of Dr. Glen Sizemore.)

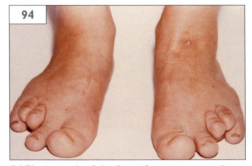

94 Photograph of the feet of a patient revealing brachydactyly of the third and fourth digits. (Courtesy of Dr. Glen Sizemore.)

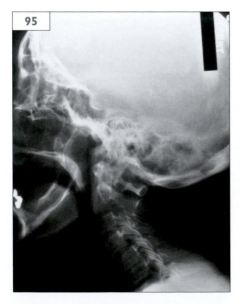

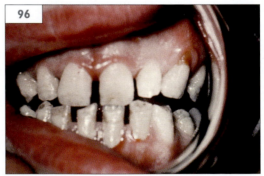

96 Dental hypoplasia in a patient with pseudohypoparathyroidism. (Courtesy of Dr. Glen Sizemore.)

95 Basal ganglia calcification of a patient with hypoparathyroidism. (Courtesy of Dr. Glen Sizemore.)

## CLINICAL PRESENTATION
The clinical findings associated with hypoparathyroidism are primarily due to the level of the serum calcium. When hypocalcemia occurs acutely, clinical manifestations include tetany, muscle cramps, muscle spasms, myopathy, paresthesias, seizures, fatigue, anxiety, and lethargy. When the hypocalcemia occurs more chronically, patients may have very few symptoms apart from the history of cataracts. The examination findings are also somewhat dependent upon the degree and duration of hypoglycemia. Findings include hypotension, a positive Trosseau's sign (carpal spasm with inflation of the blood pressure cuff above systolic), a positive Chvosteks' sign (facial muscle contraction when the facial nerve is tapped on the ipsilateral side anterior to the ear), papilledema, congestive heart failure, dry and coarse skin and hair, and brittle hair and nails.

Patients with pseudohypoparathyroidism present with the findings of hypoparathyroidism. Some patients will also display the clinical findings of short stature, rounded face, foreshortened fourth metacarpals, obesity, and subcutaneous calcifications characteristic of Albright's hereditary osteodystrophy.

## DIFFERENTIAL DIAGNOSIS
The differential diagnosis of hypoparathyroidism includes iatrogenic from neck surgery, infiltration of the parathyroid as seen in hemochromatosis, Wilson's disease, granulomas, or metastatic cancer, idiopathic, human immunodeficiency virus (HIV) infection, hypomagnesemia, and acute severe hypermagnesemia.

## DIAGNOSIS
Hypoparathyroidism is diagnosed on the basis of biochemical tests. In hypoparathyroidism, serum calcium concentrations are decreased and serum phosphate levels are increased. Serum PTH is inappropriately normal, low, or undetectable. Usually, serum 1,25-dihydroxy vitamin D is low. Alkaline phosphatase activity is normal. Intestinal calcium absorption and bone resorption are both suppressed. The renal filtered load of calcium is decreased, and the 24-hour urinary calcium excretion is reduced. Renal tubular reabsorption of phosphate is elevated. A bone densitometry scan in patients with chronic hypoparathyroidism shows defects in the mineralization of new bone. In pseudohypoparathyroidism, diagnosis generally is made on the basis of the measurement of low cAMP and phosphate levels in the urine following an infusion of synthetic PTH (1-34). The exception is in pseudohypoparathyroidism type 2 in which there is a normal increase in cAMP levels in response to synthetic PTH, but no phosphaturic response.

## MANAGEMENT/TREATMENT
Treatment for hypoparathyroidism includes therapies targeted to the underlying cause when possible, as well as the normalization of the serum calcium level. Calcium salts, 1,25-dihydroxy vitamin D, vitamin D analogs, and magnesium are the mainstay of therapy. For patients with symptoms such as seizures, tetany, and electrocardiographic changes, as well as those in whom hypocalcemia develops suddenly, intravenous calcium should be administered. Calcium gluconate is preferred and should be continued until the patient is stabilized. Oral treatment with calcium salts is directed to maintain the serum calcium in the low normal range. In patients with hypoparathyroidism the PTH-dependent renal production of 1,25-dyhydroxyvitamin D is impaired. Therefore, patients require supplementation with calcitriol. Lastly, hypomagnesemia can contribute to hypoparathyroidism. Therefore, in patients with hypoparathyroidism, hypomagnesemia, and normal renal function, magnesium replacement should be initiated. Patients with hypoparathyroidism have been treated successfully with recombinant human PTH (1-34); however, the duration of effect is short lived and the drug needs to be administered subcutaneously twice daily. This drug is now currently approved only for use in the treatment of osteoporosis.

Treatment of pseudohypoparathyroidism is similar to that of hypoparathyroidism, and consists largely of calcium replacement and calcitriol. Requirements for vitamin D supplementation are usually lower than in patients with hypoparathyroidism. Supplementation with 1,25-dihydroxyvitamin D is ideal, but patients can be treated with vitamin D analogs as well. Patients with AHO may require specific treatment for problems related to their developmental and skeletal abnormalities. Patients with pseudohypoparathyroidism type 1a may require therapy for associated hypogonadism or hypothyroidism.

# Paget's disease

## DEFINITION/OVERVIEW

Paget's disease is a metabolic disorder of the bone featuring aggressive osteoclast-mediated bone resorption and impaired osteoblast-mediated bone formation, resulting in deranged skeletal remodeling causing pain, deformities, and fractures.

## ETIOLOGY

The estimated prevalence of Paget's disease in the world is about 1%. It occurs most commonly in the countries of Great Britain, Australia, New Zealand, North America, and Western Europe, where there is a prevalence of about 3%. Some studies suggest that there is a slight male preponderance. It rarely occurs in individuals under the age of 20. The exact etiology of Paget's disease is currently unknown. Family history of Paget's disease is identified in 5–40% of patients, suggesting a possible genetic component. Heterozygous mutations affecting either of two genes have been shown in affected families to be linked to Paget's disease. The first group consists of 11 different mutations, all of which are clustered around the ubiquitin-binding domain of the sequestosome 1 protein. This protein modulates activity of the NF-κβ pathway, an important mediator of osteoclast function. The second group of mutations consists of domain-specific defects within valosin-containing protein that predispose to Paget's disease in a rare syndrome also associated with late onset inclusion body myopathy and dementia. Further evidence of the heterogeneity of the genetics of Paget's disease has come from studies reporting linkage of the disease with candidate loci at chromosome 5q31, chromosome 2, and chromosome 10. Once the genes associated with these loci are identified, a fuller understanding of the pathogenesis of familial Paget's disease should follow.

Another possible etiology for Paget's disease comes from observational studies that suggest the involvement of virus particles. Particles resembling paramyxovirus nucleocapsids, as well as antigens and nucleic acid sequences of measles virus, canine distemper virus, and respiratory syncytial virus have been identified in the nuclei and cytoplasm of pagetic osteoclasts.

## PATHOPHYSIOLOGY

Paget's disease occurs as a result of overactive osteoclasts and coupled increase in osteoblastic function in a focal manner (**97**). The woven bone that is formed at a fast rate is structurally weaker and is abnormal. It typically involves just one bone or a few bones. The bones most often involved include the skull, pelvis, vertebra, femur, or tibia. Osteolytic fronts progress approximately 1 cm yearly. Subsequent 'mixed stage' disease features cortical thickening, disorganized coarse trabeculae, and bone expansion. In cases of advanced disease, bones are widened and heterogeneously ossified. This pagetic process does not spread spontaneously to adjacent bones. However, there currently is no cure.

## CLINICAL PRESENTATION

Paget's disease is usually asymptomatic and is discovered incidentally. The prevalence of the signs and symptoms of Paget's disease are

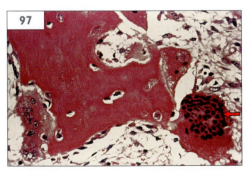

**97** Hematoxylin and eosin decalcified stained section from a bone biopsy revealing an active lesion of Paget's disease with large multinucleated osteoclasts as well as osteoblasts that are repairing bone previously resorbed by the osteoclasts. The arrow points to a giant osteoclast. (Courtesy of Dr. Glen Sizemore.)

uncertain, but the disease usually manifests itself in the skeleton. If the disease involves the skull, jaw, clavicle, or a long bone of the leg then skeletal expansion or distortion may be obvious. Mild to moderate, deep, aching bone pain characteristically begins late in the clinical course, persists throughout the day and at rest, and seems worse at night. Weight bearing often intensifies the pain especially if there are osteolytic lesions. Sudden fracture, a new mass, or constant or worsening bone pain may herald malignant transformation. Osteosarcomas, or other skeletal sarcomas, develop in less than 1% of patients with Paget's disease but are more common and aggressive than in age-matched controls. Several neurologic findings may be present. Hearing loss may result from skull involvement. Less commonly basilar impression, hydrocephalus with headache and dizziness, and cranial nerve deficits may occur. In the spine, compression or ischemia may cause pain, dysesthesias, or paralysis.

## DIFFERENTIAL DIAGNOSIS

The differential diagnosis includes Paget's disease, bone metastases, fibrous dysplasia, renal osteodystrophy, flourosis, mastocytosis, tuberous sclerosis, and osteomalacia.

## DIAGNOSIS

Paget's disease is generally diagnosed using biochemical tests. Elevated serum total or bone-specific alkaline phosphatase levels are present in patients with Paget's disease and reflect increased bone formation. Other less specific markers of bone formation include osteocalcin. Markers of bone resorption such as serum and urinary c-telopeptide and n-telopeptide are elevated in Paget's disease. The disease can be confirmed using radiographs and bone scans. The radiographic features of Paget's disease include osteolytic, osteo-sclerotic, and mixed lesions.

Histologically Paget's disease can be divided into two phases. The active phase features disorganized bone architecture. There are clusters of numerous, large, multinucleated osteoclasts adjacent to many osteoblasts. The osteoblasts synthesize matrix so rapidly that collagen forms an immature woven or lamellar pattern with faint cement lines. The stroma is vascular and fibrous. The late phase features thick trabeculae with a mosaic pattern of prominent cement lines at the interfaces of the numerous past episodes of bone resorption followed by bone formation (**98**). Osteoblast activity remains apparent with pale osteoid deposition.

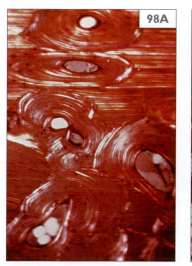 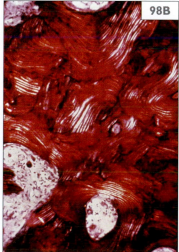

**98** Polarized views of normal bone (**A**) and Pagetic bone (**B**). The normal bone has a highly organized lamellar structure whereas the Pagetic bone displays a chaotic picture of lamellar and woven bone with disorganized structure often termed the mosaic pattern. (Courtesy of Dr. Glen Sizemore.)

Radiographs of affected areas show cortical thickening and irregular areas of lucency and sclerosis (**99, 100**). Skull involvement in Paget's disease is characterized by bony enlargement as well as cotton wool areas (**101, 102**). Involvement of the long bones often results in bowing deformities (**103, 104**). On a plain radiograph, the leading edge of an

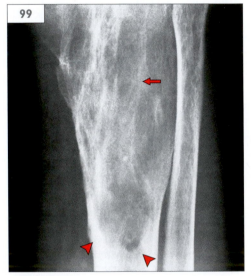

**99** Radiograph of the tibia and fibula of a patient with Paget's disease revealing an area of severe osteolytic activity (arrow) associated with a small degree of bony expansion in the distal region of the tibia (arrowheads). (Courtesy of Dr. Glen Sizemore.)

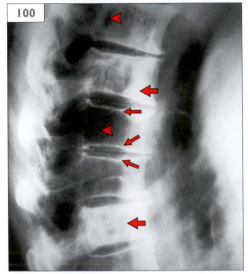

**100** Radiograph of the lateral spine of a patient with Paget's disease revealing cortical thickening (small arrows) and irregular areas of lucency (arrowheads) and sclerosis (large arrows). (Courtesy of Dr. Glen Sizemore.)

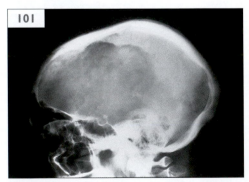

**101** Radiograph of the skull showing Paget's disease as characterized by a large circumscribed area of bone loss termed osteoporosis circumscripta, a common finding in Paget's disease. (Courtesy of Dr. Glen Sizemore.)

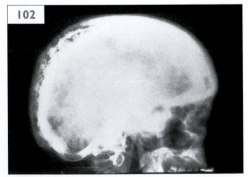

**102** Radiograph of the skull showing the late sclerotic phase of Paget's disease as characterized by tremendous thickening of the cranial vault with chaotic bone structure. (Courtesy of Dr. Glen Sizemore.)

osteolytic front in the appendicular bones often appears shaped like a flame, a letter V, or a blade of grass (**105**). Bone scans in patients with Paget's disease reveal intense uptake at pagetic areas. Usually the bone scan reveals lesions throughout the body particularly in areas such as the pelvis, vertebra, and scapula (**106**).

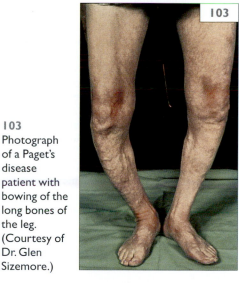

**103**
Photograph of a Paget's disease patient with bowing of the long bones of the leg. (Courtesy of Dr. Glen Sizemore.)

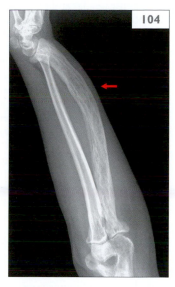

**104**
Radiograph of the arm in a patient with Paget's disease revealing bowing of the radius as well as cortical thickening and irregular areas of lucency and sclerosis (arrow).

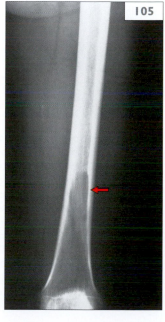

**105**
Radiograph of a long bone in a patient with Paget's disease showing the leading edge of an osteolytic front appearing shaped like a flame, a letter V, or a blade of grass. (Courtesy of Dr. Glen Sizemore.)

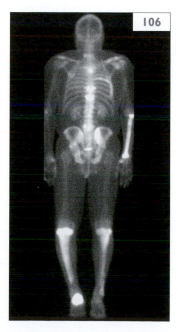

**106** Bone scan of patient with Paget's disease revealing lesions throughout the body particularly in areas such as the pelvis, vertebra, long bones, and scapula.

## MANAGEMENT/TREATMENT

There is no cure for Paget's disease. The severity of the disease is variable. Morbidity and mortality come from the pain, deformity, fracture, and sarcomatous degeneration of pagetic bone. The goal of therapy is to slow osteoclastic bone resorption. There are several indications for treatment of patients with Paget's disease. Treat if (1) the serum alkaline phosphatase is at least three or four times the upper limit of normal; (2) there are fractures or pain in the pagetic bone; (3) if there is skull involvement with hearing loss or headaches; (4) monostotic disease of weight bearing bones; (5) if there is involvement of critical sites that may lead to complications such as arthritis or fractures; and (6) in order to pretreat patients prior to surgery to reduce hypervascularity and blood loss.

The most commonly used agents for the treatment of Paget's disease are the bisphosphonates. These agents are synthetic analogs of inorganic pyrophosphate that are not biodegradable. They have skeletal half-lives measured in years, and adhere to mineralized surfaces. Osteoclasts selectively take up bisphosphonates resulting in the disruption of energy metabolism and specific enzymatic pathways. Both the oral and intravenous agents have been proven effective, with intravenous zoledronic acid showing superior response rate and longer duration of remission. After a first course of treatment, these agents are able to normalize markers of bone turnover in most patients with moderate to severe Paget's disease. Furthermore, most patients report relief of pain. After a single course, biochemical remission can persist for 6–18 months with the oral bisphosphonates and several years with zoledronic acid. A major side-effect of oral bisphosphonates is upper gastrointestinal irritation.

Intravenous pamidronate or zoledronic acid avoids this side-effect, but after an infusion patients may complain of transient mild fever, myalgias, headache, and malaise that are responsive to analgesics and antipyretics. This, however, is uncommon and is not seen in more than 15% of patients. Transient iritis develops in some patients treated with intravenous pamidronate. With all bisphosphonates there is a risk for osteonecrosis of the jaw.

Paget's disease can be treated with subcutaneous calcitonin as a second-line agent. Treatment with calcitonin remains an option if bisphosphonates are not tolerated or contraindicated. Calcitonin has been shown to decrease markers of bone turnover by 50%. It also often decreases bone pain and warmth, improves neurologic complications, and can heal osteolytic lesions. One drawback is that soon after cessation of therapy disease reactivation is likely. About 25% of patients acquire resistance to calcitonin. Side-effects include nausea and flushing.

## Osteomalacia

### DEFINITION/OVERVIEW

Osteomalacia is a term that encompasses several disorders all of which are characterized by defective bone matrix mineralization. The term rickets is often used interchangeably with osteomalacia. Rickets generally refers to defective bone matrix mineralization of the newly formed bone and growth plate cartilage present in children. Osteomalacia generally refers to defective bone matrix mineralization at the sites of bone remodeling present in both children and adults.

### ETIOLOGY

The prevalence of osteomalacia is dependent upon the criteria used for diagnosis, i.e. clinical, biochemical, bone histology, or quantitative bone histomorphometry. In studies describing bone histomorphometry of the femoral head or iliac crest biopsy in patients with hip fracture, the frequency of osteomalacia was shown to range from none to more than 30%. Defective bone matrix mineralization can be caused by: (1) calcium deficiency (hypocalcemic osteomalacia); (2) phosphorous deficiency (hypophosphatemic osteomalacia); or (3) primary defects in local bone processes (osteomalacia with normal mineral homeo-stasis). Hypocalcemic osteomalacia is essentially due to vitamin D deficiency. Vitamin D deficiency can occur as a result of inadequate nutritional intake, lack of exposure to sunlight, and intestinal malabsorption syndromes such as celiac sprue or inflammatory bowel disease.

Pseudovitamin D deficiency has also been described. It consists of two syndromes caused by congenital errors in vitamin D metabolism. Pseudovitamin D deficiency type I is an autosomal recessive disorder resulting in a defect in renal tubular 25(OH)D-1-alpha hydroxylase and thereby 1,25-dihydroxy-vitamin D deficiency. Pseudovitamin D deficiency type II is a hereditary condition resulting in defects in the calcitriol receptor effector system leading to resistance to 1,25-dihydroxyvitamin D.

Hypophosphatemic rickets is an X-linked disorder that results in decreased renal tubular absorption of phosphorus. The disease affects males and is characterized by hypophos-phatemia, growth retardation, and lower limb deformities. A milder case can occur in females who are heterozygous for the gene. Osteomalacia with normal mineral homeostasis is seen in hypophosphatasia. This rare disorder results from decreased tissue-specific alkaline phosphatase activity. Clinical presentation can vary and is generally more severe during childhood than adulthood. Hypophosphatasia is characterized by low alkaline phosphatase levels, and normal or high calcium and phosphate levels, and high serum pyridoxal 5′-phosphate.

## PATHOPHYSIOLOGY

Vitamin D derived from endogenous production in the skin or absorbed from the gut is a prohormone. It is transformed into its active form by two successive steps: hydroxylation in the liver to 25-hydroxyvitamin D followed by 1α-hydroxylation in the renal proximal tubule to 1,25-dihydroxyvitamin D. The 25-hydroxylation of vitamin D in the liver is not tightly regulated. The principal determinant of the rate of 25-hydroxylation is the circulating level of vitamin D. In contrast, the renal 1α-hydroxylase enzyme is under tight regulation by PTH, calcitonin, 1,25-dihydroxyvitamin D, calcium, and phosphorus. Once in its active form, the effects of 1,25-dihydroxyvitamin D are mediated via a high-affinity intracellular vitamin D receptor. The vitamin D receptor acts as a ligand modulated transcription factor that belongs to the steroid, thyroid, and retinoic acid receptors gene family.

1,25-dihydroxyvitamin D is the most powerful physiologic agent that stimulates active transport of calcium, and to a lesser degree phosphorus and magnesium, across the small intestine. Disorders in vitamin D action result in a decrease in the net flux of mineral to the extracellular compartment causing hypo-calcemia and secondary hyperparathyroidism. Increased renal phosphate clearance due to secondary hyperparathyroidism and reduced absorption of phosphorus due to deficient 1,25-dihydroxyvitamin D action on the gut result in hypophosphatemia. Low concen-trations of calcium and phosphorus in the extracellular fluid lead to defective mineralization of organic bone matrix.

## CLINICAL PRESENTATION

The clinical features of rickets are weakness, bone pain, bone deformity, and fracture. The most rapidly growing bones show the most striking abnormalities. Thus, the clinical features will depend on the age of onset. Rickets is not present at birth as calcium and phosphorous levels in fetal plasma are sustained by placental transport from maternal plasma that is not regulated by the fetal vitamin D system. Children with hereditary disorders of vitamin D action usually develop the characteristic features of rickets within the first 2 years of life. The rib cage may be so deformed that it contributes to respiratory failure. Dental eruption is delayed. Muscle weakness and hypotonia are severe and result in a protuberant abdomen, may contribute to respiratory failure, and may cause inability to walk without support. After the first year of life with the acquisition of erect posture and rapid linear growth, the deformities are most severe in the legs.

The clinical features of osteomalacia are subtle and may include bone pain or low back pain of varying severity. Severe muscle weakness and hypotonia may be a prominent feature in adults with osteomalacia. Improvement of myopathy occurs after very low doses of 1,25-dihydroxyvitamin D. The first clinical presen-tation of osteomalacia may be an acute fracture of the long bones, pubic ramii, ribs, or spine.

In patients with rickets occurring before the age of 2 years, physical examination often reveals widened cranial sutures, frontal bossing, posterior flattening of the skull, widening of the wrists, bulging of costochondral junction, and indentation of the ribs at the diaphragmatic insertion. The teeth usually show enamel hypoplasia. Bow legs and knock knee deformities as well as widening of the end of long bones develop as the patient becomes weight bearing. Examination findings of patients with osteomalacia are often more subtle. Patients often have bone pain, muscle weakness, hypotonia, and fractures.

## DIFFERENTIAL DIAGNOSIS

The differential diagnosis includes osteoporosis, vitamin D deficiency, liver disease, renal disease, 1-alpha hydroxylase deficiency, vitamin D resistance, X-linked hypophosphatemic rickets, autosomal dominant hypophosphatemic rickets, renal phosphate loss, excessive antacid intake, hereditary hypophosphatic rickets with hypercalciuria, drug toxicities including anticonvulsants, cholestyramine, glucocorticoids, fluoride, etidronate, parenteral aluminum, imatinab, hypophosphatasia, acidosis, and oncogenic osteomalacia.

## DIAGNOSIS

Diagnosis is primarily made through biochemical evaluation. The underlying cause can usually be determined by measuring the 25-hydroxyvitamin D, 1,25-dihydroxyvitamin D, serum calcium, 24-hour urinary calcium, serum phosphorus, intact PTH, urinary cAMP, urinary phosphate, bone-specific alkaline phosphatase, and osteocalcin. The characteristic biochemical features of vitamin D deficiency are low to low normal concentrations of serum calcium, low urinary calcium excretion, hypophosphatemia, increased serum intact PTH levels, increased urinary cAMP excretion, and decreased tubular reabsorption of phosphate. Biochemical markers associated with increased osteoid production such as bone-specific alkaline phosphatase and osteocalcin will be elevated in states of rickets and osteomalacia. If unable to make a definitive diagnosis based upon the clinical and biochemical evaluation, then the most reliable way to establish the diagnosis is with an undecalcified bone biopsy.

The characteristic histologic feature of rickets and osteomalacia is deficiency or lack of mineralization of bone matrix (**107**). In clinical practice the bone specimen obtained is from the iliac crest. Therefore, the histologic picture is osteomalacia. Osteomalacia is defined as excess osteoid and a quantitative dynamic proof of defective bone matrix mineralization obtained by analysis of time-spaced tetracycline labeling.

The specific radiographic features of rickets reflect the failure of cartilage calcification and endochondral ossification and, therefore, are best seen in the metaphyses of rapidly growing bones. The metaphyses are widened, uneven, concave, or cupped and because of the delay in or absence of calcification, the metaphyses become partially or totally invisible (**108–110**). In more severe forms, rarefaction and thinning

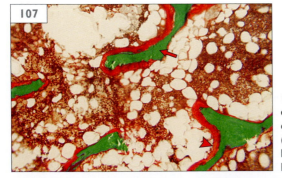

**107** Bone biopsy revealing osteomalacia as defined as excess osteoid (arrow) and defective bone matrix mineralization (arrowhead). (Courtesy of Dr. Susan Ott, http://courses.washington.edu/bonephys/op home.html.)

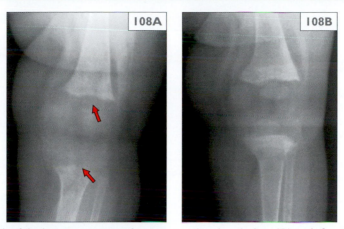

108 Radiograph of the lower extremity of a patient with rickets before (**A**), and after (**B**), treatment. The metaphyses are widened, uneven, concave, or cupped and partially invisible (arrows). (Courtesy of Dr. Glen Sizemore.)

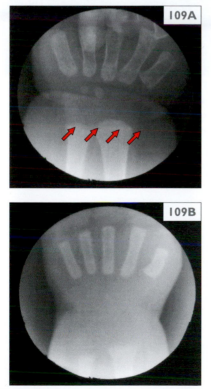

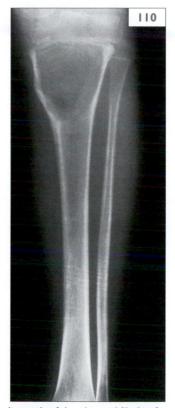

109 Radiograph of the hand of a patient with rickets before (**A**), and after (**B**), treatment. The metaphyses are widened, uneven, concave, or cupped and partially invisible (arrows). (Courtesy of Dr. Glen Sizemore.)

110 Radiograph of the tibia and fibula of a patient with rickets. The metaphyses are widened, uneven, concave, or cupped and partially invisible. (Courtesy of Dr. Glen Sizemore.)

of the cortex of the entire shaft, sparse bone trabecularization, and bone deformities will become evident. Greenstick fractures may appear as well. The radiographic features of osteomalacia are either mild, such as generalized, nonspecific osteopenia or more specific, such as pseudofractures, commonly seen at the medial edges of long bones shaft (**111**). In hypocalcemic osteomalacia, radiographic features of secondary hyperparathyroidism, such as subperiosteal resorption and cysts of the long bones, may exist.

## MANAGEMENT/TREATMENT

Rickets and osteomalacia comprise a spectrum of disease. Prognosis is dependent upon age at presentation and the severity of the disease. Patients with rickets often have lifelong morbidity and mortality. In contrast, patients with asymptomatic osteomalacia in adulthood may have a complete resolution of disease with treatment. Treatment depends in large part on the etiology of the osteomalacia. Typically, treatment consists of replacement of vitamin D with ergocalciferol, cholecalciferol or, in severe cases, calcitriol. Because vitamin D is stored in fat and released slowly and the half-life of 25-hydroxyvitamin D is 2–3 weeks, the vitamin can be given orally once a month, once every 6–12 months, or once a year by injection. Calcitriol (1,25-dihydroxyvitamin D) is given in cases where there is impaired renal conversion of 25-hydroxyvitamin D to 1,25-dihydroxyvitamin D, such as in 1-alpha hydroxylase deficiency or when there is severe malabsorption and secondary hyperparathyroidism. Patients with hypophosphatemic rickets benefit from treatment with phosphorus and 1,25-dihdroxy-vitamin D. In the case of drug-induced osteomalacia, treatment is discontinuation of the offending agent.

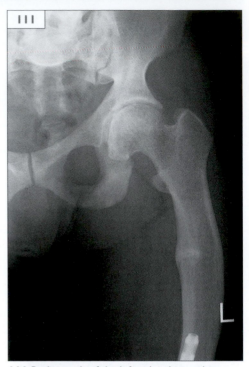

**111** Radiograph of the left pelvis, hip, and proximal half of the lower extremity with a pseudofracture at the medial edges of the femur. (Courtesy of Dr. Glen Sizemore.)

# Sclerotic bone disorders

## DEFINITION/OVERVIEW

Sclerotic bone disorders consist of a group of illnesses characterized by impaired osteoclast resorption and/or increased osteoblast-mediated bone formation, ultimately resulting in thickening of cortical and lamellar bone.

## EPIDEMIOLOGY AND ETIOLOGY

Osteopetroses are a heterogeneous group of sclerotic bone disorders defined by defects in proteins in differentiated osteoclasts, resulting in impaired osteoclast resorption. They are rare and can be grouped into three main variants: (1) the autosomal dominant benign form that occurs in adulthood termed osteopetrosis tarda; (2) the autosomal recessive malignant form that occurs in infancy termed osteopetrosis congenita; and (3) the autosomal recessive intermediate form that occurs in childhood termed marble bone disease.

Sclerotic bone disease also occurs as a consequence of prostate and breast cancer bone metastases that induce increased osteoblast activity. Bone metastases occur in up to 70 % of patients with advanced breast or prostate cancer. The exact incidence of bone metastasis is unknown, but it is estimated that 350 000 people die with bone metastases annually in the United States. Metastases to the bone are a poor prognostic sign as only 20% of patients with breast cancer are still alive 5 years after the discovery of bone metastasis.

## PATHOPHYSIOLOGY

Osteopetrosis is characterized by impaired osteoclastic bone resorption. The osteoclast is a multinucleated cell with a typical ruffled border that is capable of breaking down both the inorganic and organic matrix of bone. Osteoclastic bone resorption requires the establishment of a pH gradient across the ruffled membrane and the synthesis and release of lysosomal enzymes, in particular tartrate resistant acid phosphatase (TRAP) and cysteine proteinases such as the cathepsins, which are capable of degrading collagen. Multiple genes have been shown to be involved in the etiology and pathophysiology of osteopetrosis. The gene mutations range from autosomal recessive to autosomal dominant. The severity of the mutations ranges from moderate to malignant. It should be noted that a substantial percentage of patients with osteopetrosis have no identifiable gene defect.

The mechanisms of osteoblastic metastasis and the factors involved are unknown. Endothelin-1 has been implicated in osteoblastic metastasis from breast cancer. It stimulates the formation of bone and the proliferation of osteoblasts in bone organ cultures, and serum endothelin-1 levels are increased in patients with osteoblastic metastasis from prostate cancer. In addition to endothelin-1, platelet-derived growth factor, a polypeptide produced by osteoblasts in the bone microenvironment, urokinase, and prostate-specific antigen (PSA) may also be involved. Prostate cancer cells also release PSA, a kallikrein serine protease. PSA can cleave PTH-related peptide at the N-terminus, which could block tumor-induced bone resorption. It may also activate osteoblastic growth factors released in the bone microenvironment during the development of bone metastases.

## CLINICAL PRESENTATION

Clinical history in sclerotic bone disease is dependent upon the etiology. Autosomal recessive osteopetrosis presents in infancy and is associated with failure to thrive and growth retardation. This form of osteopetrosis is very severe and usually results in death by age 2 years. Proptosis, blindness, deafness, and hydrocephalus occur in these patients as bone encroaches on the cranial foramin. A critical feature of autosomal recessive osteopetrosis is severe bone marrow failure resulting in pancytopenia. Thrombocytopenia, leukoery-throblastic anemia, and elevated serum acid and alkaline phosphatase levels are also usually present. Hypocalcemia may or may not be present. Death from autosomal recessive osteopetrosis occurs as a result of severe anemia, bleeding, and/or infection. In rare instances patients survive into adulthood. They present with severe anemia, recurrent fractures, growth retardation, deafness, blindness, and massive hepatosplenomegaly.

Intermediate autosomal recessive osteopetrosis is not characterized by bone marrow failure and survival rates are better. Patients are usually of short stature and present with intracranial calcifications, sensorineural hearing loss, and psychomotor retardation.

Autosomal dominant osteopetrosis is asymptomatic in about 50% of cases and detected by a family history of bone disease or as an incidental radiologic finding. About 40% of patients present with fractures related to brittle osteopetrotic bones or with osteomyelitis, especially of the mandible. There is sufficient retention of marrow cavity for normal hematopoiesis to occur in patients with autosomal dominant osteopetrosis.

The consequences of bone metastases are often devastating. Patients with osteoblastic metastases have bone pain and pathologic fractures because of the poor quality of bone produced by the osteoblasts.

## DIFFERENTIAL DIAGNOSIS

The differential diagnosis of sclerotic bone disease includes malignant autosomal recessive osteopetrosis, intermediate autosomal recessive osteopetrosis, autosomal dominant osteopetrosis, severe osteoclast poor osteopetrosis, transient infantile osteopetrosis, osteopetrosis with renal tubular acidosis, osteopetrosis with neuronal anomalies, osteopetrosis with anhidrotic ectodermal dysplasia, immunodeficiency, and lymphedema, osteopetrosis with Glanzmann's thrombasthenia, and metastatic breast or prostate cancer.

## DIAGNOSIS

The diagnosis of sclerotic bone disease is derived from a combination of clinical findings, as well as radiologic evidence of dense, deformed, and diffusely sclerotic bone. Generalized osteosclerosis is apparent radiographically, often with a 'bone within a bone' appearance (**112**).

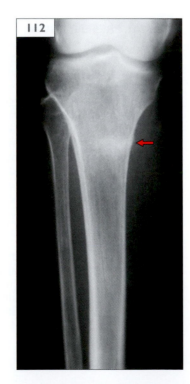

**112** Radiograph of the tibia with a sclerotic pseudofracture (arrow) as well as the typical 'bone within a bone' appearance. (Courtesy of Dr. Glen Sizemore.)

Transverse radiolucent bands may be observed, and it may be difficult to discern the marrow cavity. The decrease in osteoclast activity also affects the shape and structure of bone by altering its capacity to remodel during growth (**113**). In severely affected patients, the medullary cavity is filled with endochondral new bone, with little space remaining for hematopoietic cells. Osteosclerosis in patients with prostate or breast metastases is similar in appearance radiographically to that seen in osteopetrotic patients (**114**).

## MANAGEMENT/TREATMENT

Few therapies have proven effective in sclerotic bone disease. Bone marrow transplantation has been shown to be curative in autosomal recessive infantile osteopetrosis. It effectively treats both the bone marrow failure and the metabolic disturbances. Zoledronic acid, a potent inhibitor of osteoclast activity, differentiation, and survival, has been shown to decrease the risk of skeletal complications in males with androgen-independent prostate cancer and bone metastases. The efficacy of zoledronic acid may extend to other metastatic cancers such as metastatic breast cancer. Remaining options include treatment of associated symptoms.

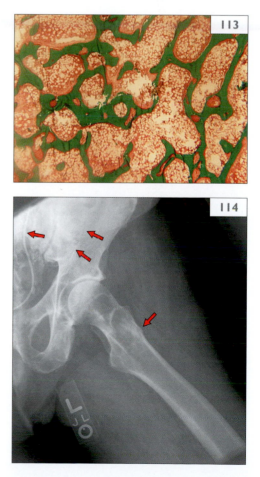

**113** Biopsy of sclerotic bone revealing increased new bone, increased disorganization, and decreased marrow cellularity. (Courtesy of Dr. Susan Ott, http://courses.washington.edu/bonephys/ophome.html.)

**114** Radiograph of the pelvis and hip revealing sclerotic osteoblastic metastatic prostate neoplasms (arrows) involving the sacrum, right and left innominate bones, and the left greater trochanter.

# Hypothalamic–pituitary disorders

S. Sethu K. Reddy

**Introduction**

**Pituitary adenomas**

**Prolactinoma**

**Acromegaly**

**Cushing disease and ectopic ACTH syndrome**

**Other pituitary adenomas**

**Pituitary apoplexy**

**Posterior pituitary**

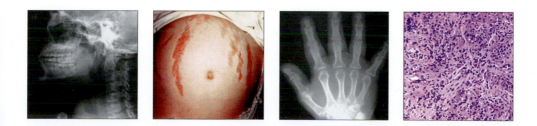

## Introduction

The pituitary gland is divided into two lobes: anterior (developed from Rathke's pouch) and posterior (developed as a diverticulum growing downward from the base of the hypothalamus). It weighs less than a gram and sits in the sella turcica which is surrounded by bony walls and floor and a roof made up of dura and then the optic chiasma, hypothalamus, and third ventricle. The optic chiasma may be anterior (15%), above (80%), or behind the sella (5%). Laterally on each side is the cavernous sinus, internal carotid artery, and cranial nerves III, IV, V1, V2, and VI.

The median eminence is an intensely vascular component at the base of the hypothalamus that forms the floor of the third ventricle. The pituitary stalk arises from the median eminence. The hypothalamus extends anteriorly to the optic chiasm and posteriorly to the mamillary bodies.

Most of the anterior pituitary hormones have associated stimulatory releasing hormones: luteinizing hormone-releasing hormone (LHRH) for both luteinizing hormone (LH) and follicle stimulating hormone (FSH); corticotrophin-releasing hormone (CRH) for adrenocorticotrophic hormone (ACTH); thyrotropin-releasing hormone (TRH) for thyroid-stimulating hormone TSH; growth hormone-releasing hormone (GHRH) for growth hormone (GH). Of note, prolactin (PRL) is under tonic inhibitory influence, with dopamine acting as a PRL release inhibiting factor (*Table 7*). Magnetic resonance imaging (MRI) is the best method for visualization of hypothalamic–pituitary anatomy, optic chiasm, vascular structures, and tumor extension to cavernous sinuses.

## Pituitary adenomas

### DEFINITION/OVERVIEW

Pituitary adenomas are tumors that may present with either hypofunction or hyperfunction, as well as symptoms directly related to mass effect (*Table 8*). Since the advent of computed tomography (CT), microadenomas have been arbitrarily designated as equal or less than 10 mm (**115** *overleaf*) in diameter and macroadenomas as greater than 10 mm in diameter (**116** *overleaf*). They are invariably benign, with no sex predilection. Pituitary adenomas are rarely associated with parathyroid and pancreatic hyperplasia or neoplasia as part of the multiple endocrine neoplasia type 1 (MEN1) syndrome. Pituitary carcinomas are rare, but metastases from other solid malignancies can occur more frequently.

Table 7  Pituitary hormones, hypothalamic hormones, and other regulatory factors

| Pituitary hormones | Hypothalamic hormones | Other regulatory factors |
| --- | --- | --- |
| Thyrotropin (TSH) | TRH | T4, T3, dopamine, Pit 1 |
| ACTH | CRH | ADH, adrenalin, cortisol |
| LH | LHRH | Estrogen, progesterone, testosterone |
| FSH | LHRH | Activin, estrogen, inhibin, follistatin, testosterone |
| GH | GHRH | Somatostatin, estrogens, T4, Pit 1 |
| PRL | PRF | Dopamine, TRH, Pit 1, estrogen, serotonin, vasoactive intestinal peptide, GnRH associated peptide |

ACTH: adrenocorticotrophic hormone; CRH: corticotrophin-releasing hormone; FSH: follicle-stimulating hormone; GH: growth hormone; GHRH: growth hormone-releasing hormone; GnRH: gonadotropin-releasing hormone; LH: luteinizing hormone; LHRH: luteinizing hormone-releasing hormone; PRF: prolactin releasing factor; PRL: prolactin; TRH: thyrotropin-releasing hormone;

Table 8  Clinical manifestations of pituitary tumors

| | Endocrine effects | |
| --- | --- | --- |
| **Mass effects** | **Hyperpituitarism** | **Hypopituitarism** |
| Headaches | GH: acromegaly | GH: short stature in children, |
| Chiasmal syndrome | PRL: hyperprolactinemia | Increased fat mass, decreased strength and well-being in adults |
| Hypothalamic syndrome | ACTH: Cushing's disease | |
| • Disturbances of thirst, appetite, satiety, sleep, and temperature regulation | Nelson's syndrome | PRL: failure of postpartum lactation |
| | LH/FSH: gonadal dysfunction or silent α-subunit secretion | ACTH: hypocortisolism |
| • Diabetes insipidus | | LH or FSH: hypogonadism |
| • SIADH | TSH: hyperthyroidism | TSH: hypothyroidism |
| Obstructive hydrocephalus | | |
| Cranial nerves III, IV, V1, V2, and VI dysfunction | | |
| Temporal lobe dysfunction Nasopharyngeal mass | | |
| • CSF rhinorrhea | | |

ACTH: adrenocorticotrophic hormone; CSF: cerebrospinal fluid; FSH: follicle-stimulating hormone; GH: growth hormone; LH: luteinizing hormone; PRL: prolactin; SIADH: syndrome of inappropriate antidiuretic hormone secretion; TSH: thyroid-stimulating hormone.

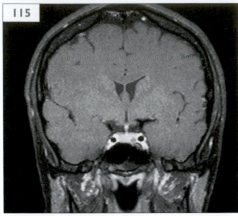

115 Pituitary microadenoma. Scan of a 40-year-old male with a 4 mm hypodense lesion in the left lateral pituitary. There was no evidence of any pituitary hypo- or hyperfunction. Pituitary adenomas tend to be hypointense on T1 and more likely to be hyperintense on T2-weighted images. With gadolinium contrast, the pituitary adenoma is initially hypointense and later hyperintense.

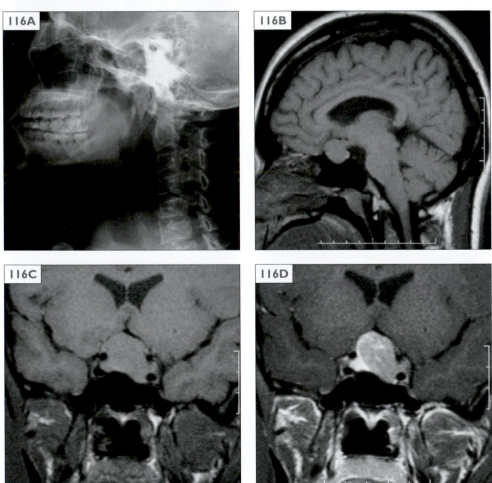

116 Pituitary macroadenoma. **A:** Abnormal eroded sella, confirmed by MRI image (**B**). The coronal images, pre- (**C**) and postcontrast (**D**) show the true extent of the tumor with evidence of wrapping around the carotid vessel.

## ETIOLOGY

About 50% of pituitary adenomas are prolactinomas, 15% GH producing (**117**), 10% ACTH-producing, and less than 1% secrete TSH. Nonfunctioning pituitary adenomas, or more appropriately named nonsecretory adenomas, represent about 25% of pituitary tumors. Most of these adenomas on morphologic examination reveal granules containing hormones, typically components of glycoprotein hormones.

Impingement on the chiasma or its branches by pituitary pathology may result in visual field defects, with the most common being bitemporal hemianopsia. Lateral extension of the pituitary mass to the cavernous sinuses may result in diplopia, ptosis, or altered facial sensation. Among the cranial nerves, third nerve palsy is the most common.

Autopsy studies suggest that up to 20% of normal individuals harbor incidental pituitary microadenomas that are pathologically similar in distribution to those that present clinically. The initial work-up should be limited and include serum prolactin and insulin-like growth factor-1 (IGF-1) level. Other screening tests may be performed depending on clinical features. The adenoma can be followed yearly by MRI, with increasing duration between imaging studies, if the size is stable.

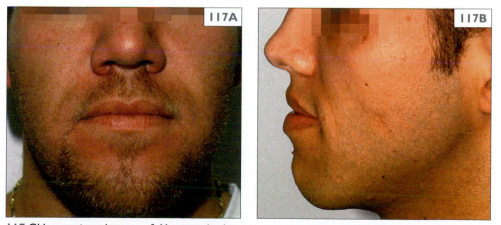

**117** GH-secreting adenoma. **A**: Young male showing some prominence of frontal sinus and prognathism of lower jaw. Of note, one should always compare with historical images to confirm a change over time. **B**: Young male demonstrating herpetegenous forehead wrinkling and prognathism.

# Prolactinoma

## DEFINITION/OVERVIEW

Hyperprolactinemia is the most common pituitary disorder. Observational studies in patients with microadenomas indicate that serum PRL concentration or adenoma size increase in only a minority of patients and, indeed, serum PRL decreases in the majority of cases over time. Estrogen therapy in the past has been suggested as a cause of prolactinoma formation, but careful case–cohort studies have found no evidence that oral contraceptives induce development of prolactinomas. Clonal analysis of tumor deoxyribonucleic acid (DNA) indicates that prolactinomas are monoclonal in origin.

## PATHOPHYSIOLOGY AND CLINICAL PRESENTATION

Hyperprolactinemia impairs pulsatile gonadotropin release (LH and FSH), likely through alteration in hypothalamic LHRH secretion. Women of reproductive age usually present with oligomenorrhea, amenorrhea, galactorrhea, and infertility. Those with long-standing amenorrhea are less likely to have galactorrhea, likely secondary to long-standing estrogen deficiency. Men and postmenopausal women usually come to medical attention because of mass effect such as headaches and visual field defects. Many men with hyperprolactinemia do not report any sexual dysfunction, but once treated effectively for hyperprolactinemia, the majority realizes the previous presence of problems including decreased libido and erectile dysfunction (*Table 9*). Men with long-standing hypogonadism may have decreased facial and body hair and soft but usually normal sized testicles (if hypogonadism starts before completion of puberty, testicles will be small). Patients with microadenomas have a higher frequency of headaches compared to control subjects.

Premenopausal women tend to present earlier with hyperprolactinemia than men or postmenopausal women. Thus, the latter often present with macroadenomas and symptoms of anterior hormone deficiency and local mass effect in the sella. Prolactinomas are four times more common in women.

**Table 9  Clinical presentation of hyperprolactinemia**

|  | Men | Women |
|---|---|---|
| **Early** |  | Irregular menses |
|  |  | Polycystic ovary syndrome |
|  |  | Reduced fertility |
|  |  | Galactorrhea |
| **Late** | Hypogonadism | Osteoporosis |
|  | Erectile dysfunction |  |
|  | Reduced energy |  |
|  | Galactorrhea |  |
|  | Headaches |  |
|  | Impaired visual field |  |
|  | Gynecomastia |  |

## DIFFERENTIAL DIAGNOSIS

It is critical to evaluate drug history carefully since some medications are associated with hyperprolactinemia and their discontinuation (if possible) will avoid any further, often expensive, work-up. Other common conditions associated with elevated PRL levels include pregnancy and hypothyroidism (*Table 10*).

## DIAGNOSIS

The PRL level usually correlates well with the size of the tumor. A serum PRL level above 200 µg/L is almost always indicative of a PRL-producing pituitary tumor. Conversely, a serum PRL level below 200 µg/L in the presence of a large pituitary adenoma is usually suggestive of stalk compression. However, one must be wary of the 'hook effect' phenomenon, which leads to modest elevations in PRL (below 200 µg/L) despite the presence of a large tumor. This occurs when extremely elevated levels of PRL interferes with the assay by saturating both the capture and signal antibodies, thus preventing binding. If suspected, the test should be repeated with 1:100 dilution of the serum. Stimulatory tests, including TRH stimulation test to determine whether an elevated PRL is a result of a prolactinoma, are nonspecific and cannot be used to diagnose or exclude a tumor.

## MANAGEMENT/TREATMENT

Medical therapy with dopamine agonists is now the first-line treatment, since surgical resection is curative only in a minority of patients and is associated with risk of recurrence in all patients. Bromocriptine mesylate, pergolide mesylate, and cabergoline are potent inhibitors of PRL secretion and often result in tumor shrinkage. Suppression of prolactin secretion by dopamine agonists depends on the number and affinity of

**Table 10 Differential diagnosis of hyperprolactinemia**

| Physiologic | Pathologic | Pharmacologic |
| --- | --- | --- |
| Pregnancy | Prolactinoma | TRH |
| Postpartum | Acromegaly (25%) | Psychotropic medications |
| Newborn | Hypothalamic disorders | Phenothiazines |
| Stress | 'Chiari–Frommel' | Reserpine |
| Hypoglycemia | Craniopharyngioma | Methyldopa |
| Sleep | Metastatic disease | Estrogen therapy |
| Postprandial hypoglycemia | Pituitary stalk secretion or compression | Metoclopramide, cimetidine (especially intravenous) |
| Intercourse | Hypothyroidism | Opiates |
| Nipple stimulation | Renal failure | Verapamil |
| | Liver disease | Some of SSRI including fluoxetine and fluvoxamine |
| | Chest wall trauma (burns, shingles) | |

SSRI: selective serotonin reuptake inhibitor; TRH: thyrotropin-releasing hormone.

dopamine receptors on lactotrope adenoma. There is usually a substantial decrease in prolactinoma size even when serum PRL levels do not normalize. These medications should be initiated slowly, since side-effects often occur at the beginning of treatment. The most common side-effects include nausea, headache, dizziness, nasal congestion, and constipation. It is important to remember that it may take up to 6 months before testosterone increases and normal sexual function is restored in men successfully treated for prolactinomas. PRL appears to have an independent effect in men on libido, since exogenous testosterone works poorly in restoring libido in those who continue to have elevated PRL levels.

While patients with microadenomas or patients without an evidence of a pituitary tumor can sometimes be followed without therapy, patients with macroadenomas always need to be treated. Occasionally, a patient with micro-adenoma or no definite pituitary tumor will have stable PRL levels after dopamine agonist discontinuation. For this reason, it would be reasonable to try a 'drug holiday' after several years of therapy with close follow-up.

Recently, an association was found between the use of dopamine agonist, pergolide and cabergoline and cardiac valve regurgitation. However, subsequent studies have shown conflicting results. The clinician needs to be aware of this possibility and order an echocardiogram if clinically suspected. Medical therapy during pregnancy often stirs debate about the continuation of bromocriptine. Tumor-related complications are seen in about 15% of pregnancies and in only 5% of women with microadenomas. A sensible approach would be to stop bromocriptine when pregnancy begins, and then follow the clinical status with MRI and visual field examinations. PRL levels may be misleading in pregnancy. If there is significant worsening in clinical status, bromocriptine could be reinstituted. A large review of over 2500 pregnancies with bromocriptine use did not reveal any increase in maternal or fetal complications related to therapy. In a follow-up study of over 900 children exposed to bromocriptine *in utero*, there were no developmental delays observed. Macropro-lactinomas are more likely to worsen during pregnancy with symptomatic growth observed in up to 40% of pregnancies. Breast-feeding has not been associated with tumor growth.

Even in the presence of mass effect symptoms such as visual field defects, dopamine agonists are the first line of therapy, since a rapid improvement in symptoms are observed in the majority of patients. Trans-sphenoidal resection is preferred and reserved for patients with disease refractory to medical therapy. The main advantage of surgery is avoidance of chronic medical therapy. Radiation therapy may be considered for patients who poorly tolerate dopamine agonists and will likely not be cured by surgery (e.g. tumor invasion of cavernous sinuses).

# Acromegaly

### DEFINITION/OVERVIEW

Acromegaly is a disease that results from excessive GH secretion usually from a pituitary tumor (**118**). It occurs at a rate of 3–4 cases per million per year with mean age at diagnosis of 40 years in males and 45 years in females.

### ETIOLOGY AND DIFFERENTIAL DIAGNOSIS

Acromegaly is caused by GH secreting pituitary tumors (95%) and, rarely, by ectopic GHRH secretion by carcinoids or pancreatic islet cell tumors. Somatotrope adenomas are monoclonal in origin. Recently, a Gsp mutation in a $Gsp_{I\alpha}$ subunit in GH cells, leading to continuous GH secretion, has been shown to result in acromegaly. Ectopic GH secretion has been documented in extracts of lung adenocarcinoma, breast and ovarian cancers; none of these conditions, except one case of pancreatic tumor, has been reported to cause acromegaly.

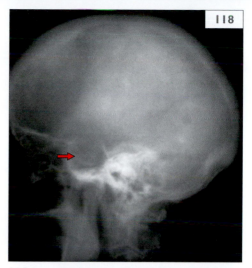

**118** Acromegaly due to a pituitary tumor. (Courtesy of Dr. Donald Gordon.)

## CLINICAL PRESENTATION

The GH-secreting tumors tend to be more aggressive in younger patients. Classic clinical features include:

- Coarsening of facial features (**119**).
- Prominent jaw and frontal sinus (**120**).
- Broadening of hands and feet (**121–123**).
- Hyperhidrosis.
- Macroglossia (**119C**).
- Signs of hypopituitarism.
- Diabetes mellitus (10–25%).
- Skin tags (screening for colonic polyps required).
- Hypertension (25–30%).
- Cardiomyopathy (50–80%).
- Carpal tunnel syndrome.
- Sleep apnea (5%).

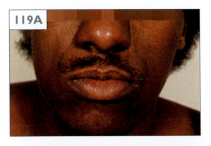

119A

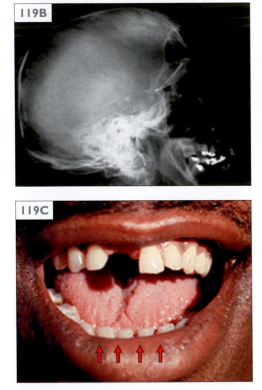

119B

119C

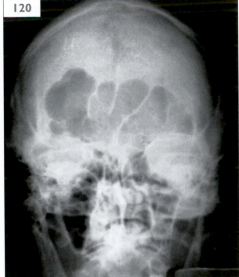

120

120 Enlarged sinuses in acromegaly. (Courtesy of Dr. Donald Gordon.)

119 Coarse facies due to bone overgrowth in acromegaly. (Courtesy of Dr. Donald Gordon.)

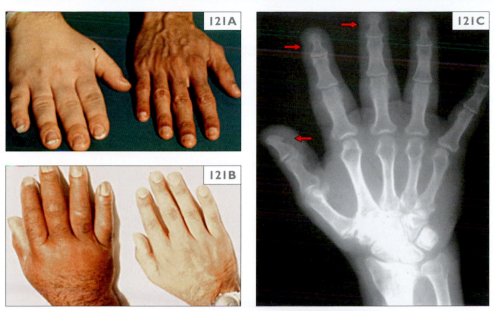

**121** Hands in acromegaly: thick fingers, spade-like hands, tufting of terminal phalanges. (Courtesy of Dr. Donald Gordon.)

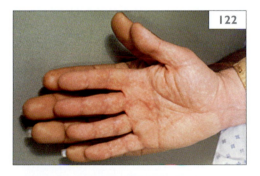

**122** Hand in acromegaly: thickening of fingers and palm. (Courtesy of Dr. Donald Gordon.)

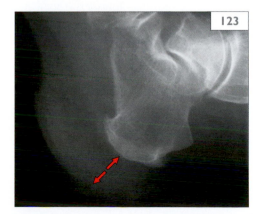

**123** Thick heel pad in acromegaly.

Other features include overgrowth of vertebrae (**124**), degenerative arthritis (**125**), and acanthosis nigricans (**126**). Particular attention to early detection of cardiovascular disease is of paramount importance. Patients with acromegaly have a 3.5-fold increased mortality rate, often due to cardiovascular disease. In addition, acremegalic patients have increased risk of colon polyps with potential for increased risk of malignancy, affecting their life expectancy. For this reason they should undergo colonoscopy every 3–5 years until more data about frequency of such screening tests are available. It is not clear if more rigorous screening for a variety of cancers including breast, lung, or prostate cancer is indicated in these patients.

## DIAGNOSIS

Random GH levels can overlap in acromegalic patients and controls, due to GH's pulsatility. Therefore, a single GH level is inadequate to establish the diagnosis. IGF-1 has a longer plasma half-life than GH and is an excellent initial screening test for those suspected to have acromegaly. An elevated IGF-1 level in a clinical setting suggestive of acromegaly almost always confirms the diagnosis. One should be aware that concomitant poorly controlled diabetes or malnutrition could be associated with low IGF-1 levels. The oral glucose tolerance test remains the gold standard test to confirm the diagnosis. Normal individuals suppress their GH level to less than 1 µg/L (using chemiluminescent assays) within 2 hours after ingestion of 100 g oral glucose solution.

In the case of ectopic acromegaly, elevated GHRH can be measured in blood to confirm the diagnosis (usually >300 ng/mL). In the rare patient with a hypothalamic GHRH-secreting tumor, peripheral GHRH levels may be normal. In patients with a GH-secreting pituitary adenoma, GHRH level is low or undetectable. About 70% of patients with acromegaly have been shown to display a paradoxical GH response to TRH but unfortunately with the lack of availability of TRH, this test is no longer easily accessible.

## MANAGEMENT/TREATMENT

The primary aims of treatment include relieving the symptoms, reducing tumor bulk, normalization of IGF-1 and GH dynamics and prevention of tumor regrowth. Medical treatment of acromegaly has improved over the last couple of decades, since the limitations of radiation and surgical therapy have become evident. Analogs of somatostatin are the most effective medical therapy available for acromegaly. Octreotide therapy has been shown to lower and normalize IGF-1 in 90% and 65% of patients, respectively. It is usually given as subcutaneous injection three times per day. The long-acting octreotide (sandostatin LAR) can be given monthly intramuscularly. Long-term observations of patients on somatostatin analogs have shown no evidence for tachyphylaxis. Some degree of tumor shrinkage in up to 50% of patients is expected, although in most cases there is less than 50% shrinkage in tumor size. The most common side-effects are gastrointestinal, including diarrhea, abdominal pain, and nausea. The most serious side-effect of sandostatin analogs is cholelithiasis, seen in up to 25% of patients. Its management is similar to those with cholelithiasis in the general population and routine ultrasonographic screening is not indicated. This type of therapy may be quite useful as an adjunct to radiotherapy since radiotherapy may take several years to reduce GH levels significantly.

Normalization of IGF-1 is seen in only 10–15% of patients treated with dopamine agonists and is more likely with pituitary tumors secreting both GH and PRL. Pegvisomant, a GH receptor antagonist is the most recent addition to the list of pharmacologic agents for acromegaly. This is administered as a daily subcutaneous injection. IGF-1 is significantly reduced and clinical symptoms improve; however, growth of the tumor is not inhibited and rare cases of tumor enlargement have been reported.

The surgical approach is the treatment of choice in those presenting with pituitary microadenomas or when the tumor is confined to sella, with a cure rate of up to 90%. For those with macroadenomas, surgical cure is observed in less than 50% of cases. Even in those not cured by surgery, tumor debulking usually results in improvement of symptoms and lowering of IGF-1 levels. Radiation therapy almost always induces a decrease in size of the tumor and GH level, but often fails to normalize IGF-1 levels. In the view of low efficacy, high risk of hypopituitarism and lack of

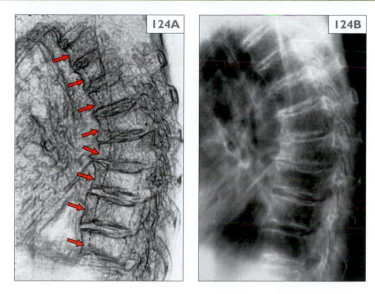

**124** Overgrowth of vertebrae in acromegaly. (Courtesy of Dr. Donald Gordon.)

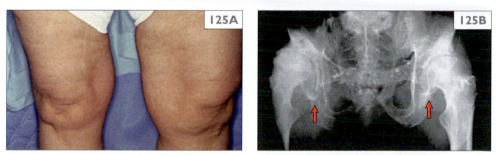

**125** Degenerative arthritis in acromegaly. (Courtesy of Dr. Donald Gordon.)

knowledge about long-term effect on neuropsychiatric functions, radiation therapy should be reserved for those not responsive to other treatment modalities. Radiosurgery (gamma knife) seems to be superior to conventional radiation therapy, but large studies with strict cure criteria including normalization of IGF-1 and long-term safety profile are lacking. GH antagonists are being currently investigated.

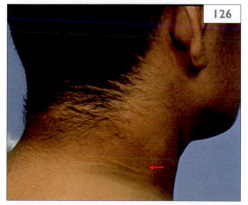

**126** Acanthosis nigricans in acromegaly. (Courtesy of Dr. Donald Gordon.)

# Cushing disease and ectopic ACTH syndrome

## DEFINITION/OVERVIEW

Cushing disease and ectopic ACTH syndrome are associated with excess cortisol secretion caused by ACTH from the pituitary or a nonpituitary tumor, respectively. ACTH-secreting pituitary adenoma is the most common cause of endogenous Cushing syndrome (CS) (60%) with the rest being adrenal (25%) or ectopic (15%) in origin (**127, 128**).

## CLINICAL PRESENTATION

The following findings are suggestive of hypercortisolism state:
- Central obesity.
- Muscle wasting with proximal muscle weakness.
- Thinning of skin and connective tissue.
- Osteopenia/osteoporosis.
- Spontaneous ecchymosis.
- Purplish wide striae (>1 cm) (**129**).
- Hypokalemia.

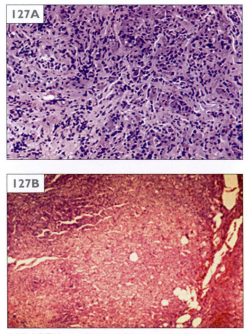

**127** ACTH-producing adenoma resulting in adrenal hyperplasia in Cushing's syndrome.

Other findings, which are less helpful in discriminating patients with and without Cushing's, are hypertension, abnormal glucose tolerance, menstrual irregularities, and psychiatric disturbances including depression. Women with Cushing's disease typically have fine facial lanugo hair and may have acne and temporal scalp hair loss secondary to increased adrenal androgen secretion. There is usually a 3–6 year delay in diagnosis of patients with Cushing's disease and it may be possible to date the onset of the disease by determining which scars are pigmented due to excess secretion of ACTH and other melanotropins.

## DIAGNOSIS

Twenty-four hour urinary free cortisol measurement is the single best test for diagnosis of CS. Because of the significant overlap between normal individuals and those with Cushing's, random serum cortisol has no role in the diagnosis of Cushing's syndrome. A 1 mg overnight dexamethasone suppression test with an morning cortisol level below 1.8 µg/dL virtually rules out the disease but has up to 40% false-positive rate. A combination of low-dose dexamethasone suppression test and CRH stimulation test has been shown to have 100% diagnostic accuracy in a NIH study. This test may have a significant value in establishing the diagnosis in those with pseudo-Cushing and elevated 24 hr urinary free cortisol. Other tests useful in establishing the diagnosis of Cushing's disease include midnight serum and salivary cortisol (**130**).

Once the diagnosis of CS has been established, the next step is to find out whether it is ACTH dependent (**130**). While undetectable or low ACTH are consistent with adrenal etiology, low normal ACTH may be seen in both ectopic Cushing and those with an ACTH-secreting pituitary tumor. CRH stimulation test is used for differentiation between the two. Although ACTH levels tend to be higher in those with ectopic CS compared to patients with pituitary disease, there is considerable overlap. High-dose dexamethasone test and/or CRH stimulation test are helpful in differentiation of the two. Cortisol levels are not suppressed with

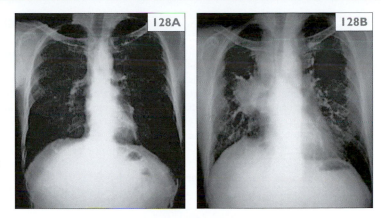

**128** Small-cell carcinoma of lung with ectopic ACTH overproduction in Cushing's syndrome.

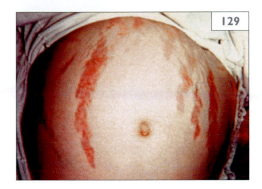

**129** Clinical features in Cushing's syndrome: purple striae.

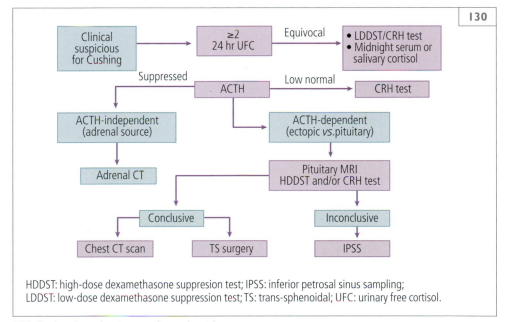

HDDST: high-dose dexamethasone suppression test; IPSS: inferior petrosal sinus sampling; LDDST: low-dose dexamethasone suppression test; TS: trans-sphenoidal; UFC: urinary free cortisol.

**130** Cushing's evaluation: work-up algorithm.

the high-dose (8 mg) dexamethasone test in patients with ectopic ACTH syndrome and CRH stimulation may not lead to a further rise in ACTH. The gold standard test to differentiate pituitary Cushing from an ectopic ACTH-producing tumor is inferior petrosal sinus sampling. This test should be performed by experienced neuroradiologist and it is essential to note that it cannot be used to make the diagnosis of Cushing's syndrome.

Ectopic ACTH syndrome is the most frequent and best studied of the ectopic hormone syndromes. Most tumors associated with ectopic ACTH syndrome are carcinomas and have a poor prognosis. They usually present as a rapid onset syndrome (within 6 months) associated with profound muscle weakness, hyperpigmentation, hypertension, hypokalemia, and edema. Hyperpigmentation is thought to be due to cosecretion of β-melanocyte stimulating hormone (β-MSH), one of the byproducts of ACTH synthesis. Some benign tumors, such as carcinoids or islet cell tumors, have been shown to cause ectopic ACTH syndrome and are difficult to differentiate from pituitary causes of Cushing's syndrome. This difficulty is exaggerated by radiologic investigations of the sella that are often negative or shows a microadenoma, which is seen in up to 20% of autopsy series in normal individuals.

## MANAGEMENT/TREATMENT

Surgical (trans-sphenoidal) removal of the ACTH-secreting pituitary tumor is the treatment of choice. Availability of an experienced surgeon is crucial with an 80–90% remission rate following surgery. An undetectable cortisol level postoperatively off steroid is considered to be an excellent marker for long-term cure. There is a period of temporary adrenal insufficiency following successful surgery, usually of 6–8 months, but may be as long as 2 years in duration. For those not cured by the surgery, other options include a second operation and radiation therapy. Patients whose tumor is unresponsive to these therapies may then be offered medical or surgical adrenalectomy. Ectopic ACTH-producing tumors should be resected if possible. Octreotide may inhibit ectopic ACTH secretion. Mitotane is perhaps the most effective adrenolytic agent. Other medications, such as aminoglutethimide, ketoconazole, or metyrapone, are useful as temporizing agents only. The investigational glucocorticoid antagonist mifepristone (RU 486, FDA approved as an antiprogesterone agent) is a promising therapy that appears to have few side-effects. One difficulty is that one cannot rely on cortisol measurements to follow the effect of mifepristone.

# Other pituitary adenomas

## Nonfunctioning or glycoprotein-secreting tumors and and TSH adenomas

### DEFINITION/OVERVIEW
Nonfunctioning or glycoprotein secreting tumors are usually clinically silent because they are inefficient in secreting hormones and lack a clinically recognizable syndrome. TSH-secreting adenomas are the most uncommonly occurring pituitary adenomas.

### CLINICAL PRESENTATION
The glycoprotein (LH or FSH) secreting adenomas usually come to attention because of manifestations of mass lesion including headache and visual field defect. Patients may present with varying degrees of hypopituitarism due to mass effect. Rarely, an FSH adenoma may cause amenorrhea in a woman, or an LH adenoma may cause precocious puberty in a boy.

The clinical picture in patients with TSH-secreting pituitary adenomas includes pituitary mass lesion, hyperthyroidism, and goiter.

### DIAGNOSIS
Diagnosis of an LH or FSH adenoma is confirmed by measurement of either intact glycoprotein hormones or their $\alpha$ and $\beta$ subunits. Levels of the $\alpha$ subunit tend to be inappropriately elevated, compared with those of the intact hormone itself. The most important biochemical feature for a TSH adenoma is elevation of thyroid hormone levels in the presence of normal or elevated TSH level. For this reason any patient presenting with endogenous hyperthyroidism and an elevated or normal TSH should be further evaluated for the presence of a TSH-secreting pituitary adenoma. Elevated serum PRL and $\alpha$ subunit are in favor of a thyrotrope adenoma and against thyroid hormone resistance syndrome.

### MANAGEMENT/TREATMENT
The trans-sphenoidal surgical approach is standard especially if visual function is abnormal. Surgery is rarely curative because of the size of adenoma on presentation, and usually radiation therapy is needed as an adjunct. Octreotide may be helpful in reducing hormone secretion but further studies are required to assess if it has any effect on tumor size. Dopamine agonists, such as bromocriptine, have been used in high doses, but clinical responses (i.e. changes in tumor size or visual symptoms) occur in less than 10% of patients. Long-acting gonadotropin-releasing hormone (GnRH) agonists and antagonists may reduce secretion of FSH and LH by tumors but do not reduce tumor size. In summary, the efficacy of the medical therapy in patients with nonfunctional or glycopreotein-secreting pituitary adenoma is not established, but is used in an attempt to reduce tumor hypersecretion and size following unsuccessful surgery.

## Lymphocytic hypophysitis

### DEFINITION/OVERVIEW
Lymphocytic hypophysitis is a disease characterized by lymphocytic infiltration of the pituitary gland which may lead to hypopituitarism.

### ETIOLOGY
The exact cause is unknown but this is likely an autoimmune phenomenon.

### PATHOPHYSIOLOGY
Lymphocytic infiltration leads to mass effect and eventually hypofunction of the pituitary.

## CLINICAL PRESENTATION

This is often seen in females during or after pregnancy. The clinical manifestations are secondary to hypopituitarism or adrenal insufficiency and/or due to a pituitary mass effect.

## DIAGNOSIS

Serum PRL is elevated in half of patients, but may be decreased. Antipituitary antibodies are present in some patients and other autoimmune endocrine disorders, including Hashimoto's thyroiditis and Addison's disease have been seen in others. MRI and CT scans of the sella reveal a pituitary mass and, in some cases, thickening of the stalk. MRI shows diffuse and homogenous contrast enhancement of the anterior pituitary area. Although the diagnosis may be suspected on clinical grounds in a pregnant or postpartum woman, surgical biopsy is needed for confirmation of the diagnosis.

## MANAGEMENT

Some patients recover fully, while others may need selective hormone replacement. For this reason, patients need to be assessed at regular intervals for the necessity of continued hormone replacement.

# Empty sella syndrome

## DEFINITION/OVERVIEW

Empty sella syndrome is often a radiologic diagnosis and is manifest by a sella which may appear to be empty to varying degrees (i.e. partial to complete) (**131, 132**).

## ETIOLOGY

While primary empty sella is the result of a congenital diaphragmatic defect, secondary empty sella may result from previous surgery, irradiation, or infarction of a pre-existing tumor.

## DIAGNOSIS

The diagnosis of the empty sella syndrome is increasingly made owing to the prevalence of CT and MRI. Pituitary fossa enlargement is secondary to communication between the pituitary fossa and subarachnoid space, which causes remodeling and enlargement of the sella. Most patients have no pituitary dysfunction, but a wide spectrum of pituitary deficiencies have been described, especially in those with secondary empty sella. Coexisting tumors may occur.

## MANAGEMENT/TREATMENT

Management is usually with reassurance and hormone replacement, if necessary. Surgery is only necessary if visual field defects occur or if there is cerebrospinal fluid rhinorrhea.

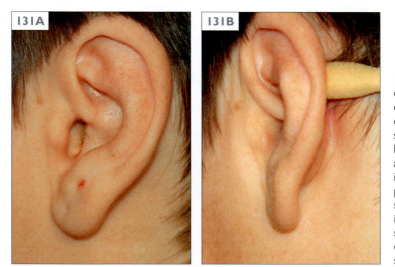

131 **A**, **B**: Images depicting auricular calcification. This clinical finding may be seen with acromegaly, hyperparathyroidism, and adrenal insufficiency. This particular subject had secondary adrenal insufficiency secondary to an empty sella syndrome.

# Hypopituitarism

### ETIOLOGY
Pituitary adenomas are the most common cause of hypopituitarism, but other causes including parasellar diseases, following pituitary surgery or radiation therapy, and head injury must also be considered. The usual consequence of pituitary hormone deficiency secondary to a mass effect is in the following order: GH, LH, FSH, TSH, ACTH, and PRL. PRL deficiency is uncommon except in those with pituitary infarction. Isolated deficiencies of various anterior pituitary hormones have also been described.

### CLINICAL PRESENTATION/ MANAGEMENT/TREATMENT OF HORMONE DEFICIENCIES
GH deficiency is now recognized as a pathologic state in adults as well as children and more patients with GH deficiency undergo GH replacement. GH deficiency may contribute to increased mortality in patients with hypopituitarism, with cardiovascular disease being the most common cause of mortality. The symptoms of GH deficiency in adults are more subtle including decreased muscle strength and exercise tolerance, and reduced sense of well-being (e.g. diminished libido, social isolation). Patients with GH deficiency have increased body fat particularly intra-abdominally and decreased lean body mass in comparison to normal adults. Some patients have decreased BMD, which may improve with GH replacement. A trial of GH replacement in adults with documented GH deficiency and symptoms or metabolic abnormalities suggestive of GH deficiency is indicated. The most common side-effects of GH therapy include fluid retention, carpal tunnel syndrome, and arthralgia. These side-effects are usually dose related and improve with dose reduction.

Gonadotropin deficiency may be secondary to a pituitary defect, hypothalamic deficiency of LHRH, or a functional abnormality such as hyperprolactinemia, anorexia nervosa, and severe disease state. In females gonadotropin deficiency causes infertility and menstrual disorders including amenorrhea. It is often associated with lack of libido and dyspareunia. In males hypogonadism is diagnosed less often, since decreased libido and impotence may be considered as a function of aging. Hypogonadism is often diagnosed retrospectively when a patient presents with mass effect. Osteopenia is a consequence of long-standing hypogonadism and usually responds to hormone replacement therapy.

The symptoms of secondary adrenal insufficiency are similar to primary adrenal insufficiency with one important difference. Mineralocorticoid secretion is mainly regulated by the renin and angiotensin system, and is preserved in patients with pituitary disorders. For this reason the symptoms are more chronic in nature, and commonly include malaise, loss of energy, and anorexia. Hyperkalemia is not a feature of secondary adrenal insufficiency. An acute illness may precipitate vascular collapse, hypoglycemia, and coma.

TSH deficiency is relatively a late finding in patients with pituitary disorders, with symptoms being similar to those with primary hypothyroidism including malaise, leg cramps, lack of energy, and cold intolerance. The degree of hypothyroidism depends on the duration of thyrotropin deficiency.

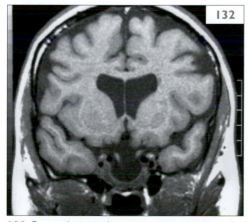

**132** Coronal image demonstrating an enlarged empty sella. Note that the intrasellar content is the same density as CSF in the lateral ventricles.

# Pituitary apoplexy

### DEFINITION/OVERVIEW
Pituitary apoplexy is an endocrine emergency resulting from hemorrhagic infarction of the pituitary, usually associated with a pre-existing pituitary tumor.

### ETIOLOGY
A variety of predisposing conditions including bleeding disorders, diabetes mellitus, pituitary radiation, pneumoencephalography (of historical interest only), mechanical ventilation, and trauma have been described.

### DIAGNOSIS
Diagnosis is made when a patient presents with classic symptoms of headache, visual disturbance, and MRI or CT shows hemorrhage within a pituitary adenoma.

### DIFFERENTIAL DIAGNOSIS
- Aneurysm of the internal carotid.
- Basilar artery occlusion.
- Hypertensive encephalopathy.
- Acute expansion of intrasellar cyst or abscess.
- Cavernous sinus thrombosis.

### CLINICAL PRESENTATION
The clinical manifestations of this syndrome is related to rapid expansion and compression of the pituitary gland and the perisellar structures leading to severe headache, hypopituitarism, visual field defects, and cranial nerve palsies. Extravasation of blood or necrotic tissue into the subarachnoid space may cause clouding of consciousness, meningismus, autonomic dysfunction, fever and, rarely, as sudden death.

Although secondary hypoadrenalism does not usually result in hypotension, acute loss of ACTH in pituitary hemorrhage can result in shock. Other deficiencies of anterior pituitary hormones may be present, but diabetes insipidus is seen only transiently in 4% of cases.

### MANAGEMENT/TREATMENT
If pituitary apoplexy is suspected, anterior pituitary insufficiency should be presumed and the patient must be treated accordingly. The glucocorticoid dose must be adequate for the degree of stress and presumptive cerebral edema. Any evidence of sudden visual field defects, oculomotor palsies, hypothalamic compression, or coma should lead to immediate surgical decompression. The recovery of a variety of pituitary hormone deficiencies following surgery have been documented and all patients should be re-evaluated for possible recovery of their pituitary hormone axes.

Sheehan's syndrome is the result of ischemic infarction of normal pituitary gland leading to hypopituitarism secondary to postpartum hemorrhage and hypotension. Patients have a history of failure to lactate postpartum, failure to resume menses, cold intolerance, or fatigue. Some women may have an acute crisis mimicking apoplexy within 30 days postpartum. There is often subclinical central diabetes insipidus (DI).

A patient with untreated hypopituitarism may decompensate acutely with stress, resulting in coma. This acute decompensation may mimic acute MI, overwhelming sepsis, a cerebrovascular accident (CVA), or meningitis. Symptoms may be a blend of acute thyroid and adrenal insufficiency. Clinical clues might consist of a myxedematous or acromegalic appearance and/or decreased body hair.

# Posterior pituitary

## INTRODUCTION

The posterior pituitary is a storage site for antidiuretic hormone (ADH, vasopressin) and oxytocin. Clinically, disorders of ADH are most relevant (*Table 11*). ADH secretion is regulated by changes in serum osmolality and/or plasma volume. Small increments in serum osmolality greater than 290 mOsm/kg lead to prompt secretion of ADH. However, more than a 10% reduction in plasma volume will override any osmolar stimulus. Pain, nicotine, and caffeine can increase ADH secretion. Native ADH is a potent vasoconstrictor but desmopressin (DDAVP), an ADH analog, has pure antidiuretic action with little vasoconstriction.

# Central diabetes insipidus

## DEFINITION/OVERVIEW

Central DI (pituitary origin) is a polyuric syndrome secondary to inadequate ADH secretion and inability to concentrate the urine. Patients have a normal response to administration of vasopressin. Maximum urine output due to complete ADH deficiency is about 18 liters per day and urine volume in excess of this indicates excess fluid intake.

## ETIOLOGY

- Familial.
- Idiopathic.
- Trauma/postsurgical.
- Granulomatous disease.
- Tumors:
  - Craniopharyngioma (**133** *overleaf*).
  - Pituitary tumors.
  - Metastatic cancer.
- Infectious.
- Vascular.
- Aneurysms.
- Sheehan's syndrome.
- Autoimmune.

Table 11 Common ADH related syndromes

| Clinical presentation | Thirst | ADH secretion | ADH action | Diagnosis |
|---|---|---|---|---|
| Polyuria/polydipsia | N | ⇓ | N | Central DI |
| Polyuria/polydipsia | N | N | ⇓ | Nephrogenic DI |
| Polyuria/polydipsia | ⇑ | N | N | Primary polydipsia |
| ⇑ Na+ | ⇓ | N | N | Hypodipsia |
| ⇓ Na+ | ⇓ | ⇑ | N | SIADH |

DI: diabetes insipidus; SIADH: syndrome of inappropriate antidiuretic hormone secretion.

## DIAGNOSIS

Patients with DI who are conscious usually have sufficient thirst to maintain a normal serum sodium in spite of polyuria. In this situation a standard water deprivation test should be performed, during which patients are allowed no fluid to drink while closely monitored. When two consecutive voided urine osmo-lalities differ by less than 30 mmol/L or when 5% of body weight is lost, 5 U of aqueous vasopressin (approximately 5 µg of DDAVP) is given intravenously with repeating urine osmolality measurements at 30 and 60 min.

Desmopressin administration following dehydration will elicit the following responses:
- Less than 9% increase in urine osmolality with maximal urine concentration during the test – normal.
- Greater than 50% rise in urine osmolality with inadequate urine concentration during the test – central DI.
- No rise in urine osmolality with inadequate urine concentration during the test – nephrogenic DI.

Serum ADH level at the end of fast and before administration of vasopressin helps to differentiate between partial central and nephrogenic DI, since both may have modest concentration of urine with dehydration and a more than 10% increase in urine osmolality in response to vasopressin.

## DIFFERENTIAL DIAGNOSIS

Patients with psychogenic polydipsia have a diluted medullary concentrating gradient and partial nephrogenic DI may develop. Some of conditions associated with nephrogenic DI include familial, tubulointerstitial renal disease, electrolytes disorder (hypokalemia and hyper-calcemia), drugs (e.g. lithium, demeclocycline), and pregnancy.

## MANAGEMENT/TREATMENT

The posterior pituitary enhances on MRI with gadolinium and is a 'good assay' of ADH reserve, keeping in mind that up to 20% of normal individuals do not have a bright spot. Partial central DI may be treated with chlorpropamide or thiazides, while complete central DI needs to be treated with desmo-pressin. The drug is available in subcutaneous, oral, and nasal spray. The exact dosing and timing have to be individualized.

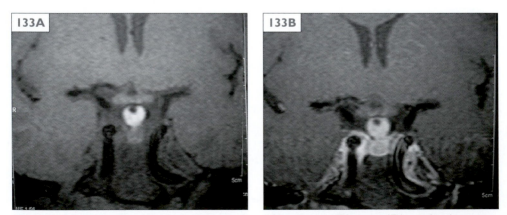

**133** Craniopharyngioma with suprasellar mass. Pre- (**A**) and post- (**B**) coronal T1-weighted images. (Courtesy of Dr. Amir Hamrahian, Endocrinology, Diabetes & Metabolism, Cleveland Clinic.)

# Adrenal disorders

Thottathil Gopan

Amir Hamrahain

**Anatomy and physiology of the adrenal gland**

**Adrenal insufficiency**

**Primary aldosteronism**

**Pheochromocytoma**

**Cushing syndrome**

**Congenital adrenal hyperplasia**

**Adrenocortical carcinoma**

**Adrenal incidentaloma**

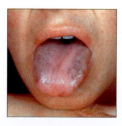 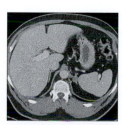 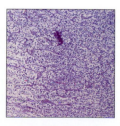 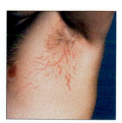

## Anatomy and physiology of the adrenal gland

The adrenal glands are paired retroperitoneal organs that lie within the perinephric fat, at the anterior, superior, and medial aspects of the kidneys. Each gland functionally consists of an outer cortex and inner medulla, which have distinct embryologic origins and produce different classes of hormones. The cortex mainly produces steroid hormones and is composed of three zones:

- The outer zona glomerulosa synthesizes aldosterone under the principal control of the renin–angiotensin system which in turn modulates both sodium and potassium homeostasis.

- The middle zona fasciculata secretes cortisol under the influence of ACTH.
- The inner zona reticularis is mostly involved in the synthesis of androgens (dehydroepiandrosterone [DHEA], dehydroepiandrosterone sulfate [DHEAS] and androstenedione).

The adrenal medulla, located in the central portion of the gland, is part of the sympathetic nervous system and produces catecholamines, mostly epinephrine.

# Adrenal insufficiency

## DEFINITION

The term 'adrenal insufficiency' (AI) refers to failure of the adrenal cortex to secrete sufficient amounts of glucocorticoids, mineralocorticoids, or both. AI can be divided into two general categories: (1) lack of adequate hormone secretion by the adrenals (primary AI) and (2) inadequate ACTH or CRH secretion (secondary AI).

## EPIDEMIOLOGY/ETIOLOGY

### Primary adrenal insufficiency

Primary AI is a rare condition with an estimated incidence in the developed world of 0.8 cases per 100 000 and a prevalence of 4–11 cases per 100 000 population. The causes of primary adrenal insufficiency are listed in *Table 12*.

Autoimmune destruction of adrenals (Addison's disease) accounts for over 70% of all cases of primary AI. About half of the patients with Addison's disease have an associated autoimmune disease, also known as autoimmune polyendocrine syndromes (APS) type I and II (please see Chapter 8 on autoimmune polyglandular failure).

Tuberculosis, fungal infections, HIV, and cytomegalovirus infection are among the most common infections associated with adrenal insufficiency. The adrenals may be involved in patients with AIDS. About 8–14% of AIDS patients demonstrate a subnormal cortisol response following a short ACTH stimulation test. Metastases from primary cancer (commonly lung and breast) usually do not cause adrenal insufficiency unless more than 90% of the adrenal glands are destroyed. Adrenal hemorrhage and adrenoleukodystrophy syndromes are other rare causes of adrenal insufficiency.

### Secondary adrenal insufficiency

Secondary AI is most often due to sudden cessation of exogenous glucocorticoid therapy. It should be anticipated in any patient who has taken more than the equivalent of 30 mg of hydrocortisone per day (7.5 mg prednisone or 0.75 mg dexamethasone) for more than 3 weeks. Other causes of secondary AI are due to deficient production of ACTH by the pituitary or CRH by the hypothalamus, and are usually accompanied by deficiencies of other pituitary hormones.

## PATHOLOGY OF AUTOIMMUNE ADRENALITIS

The pathologic changes in autoimmune adrenal insufficiency vary with the stage of the disease. In the initial stage, the adrenal glands may be enlarged, with extensive lymphocytic infiltration. In patients with long-standing disease, the adrenal glands are small and sometimes difficult to locate. The capsule is thickened and fibrotic and the cortex is completely destroyed, although there may be a few small clusters of adrenocortical cells surrounded by lymphocytes. Serum antibodies against all the three zones of the adrenal cortex are present in 60–75% of patients with autoimmune adrenalitis. The medulla is relatively spared.

## CLINICAL PRESENTATION

Patients with primary AI have both glucocorticoid and mineralocorticoid deficiency. In contrast, patients with secondary AI have an intact renin–angiotensin–aldosterone system since ACTH plays only a minor role in

**Table 12  Causes of primary adrenal insufficiency**

**Anatomic destruction of gland (acute or chronic)**

Autoimmune adrenalitis (Addison's disease)

  Autoimmune polyendocrine syndromes (APS) type I and II

Infections (tuberculosis, fungi, HIV, CMV, syphilis)

Metastatic cancer

Infiltration (e.g. amyloid)

Hemorrhage/infarction

**Metabolic failure in hormone production**

Congenital adrenal hyperplasia

Medications (ketoconazole, metyrapone, megestrol, mitotane, etomidate)

**Others**

Adrenoleukodystrophy/ adrenomyeloneuronopathy

Congenital adrenal hypoplasia

ACTH-resistant syndromes

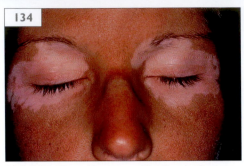

134–138 Clinical features of Addison's disease.
134 Vitiligo of the face. (Courtesy of Dr. Leann
Olansky, Department of Endocrinology,
Diabetes, and Metabolism, Cleveland Clinic.)

aldosterone secretion. Almost all patients with primary adrenal insufficiency complain of fatigue, anorexia, and weight loss. Other clinical (**134–138**) and laboratory manifestations of primary adrenal insufficiency are summarized in *Table 13*. Skin hyperpigmentation, initially on the extensor surfaces, palmar creases, and buccal mucosa results from the increased ACTH and other pro-opiomelanocortin (POMC)-related peptide production by the pituitary gland.

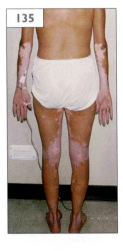

135 Vitiligo of the body. (Courtesy of Dr. Leann Olansky, Department of Endocrinology, Diabetes, and Metabolism, Cleveland Clinic.)

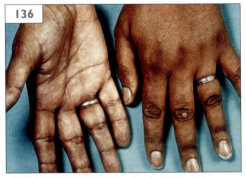

136 Hyperpigmentation of palmar creases. (Courtesy of Dr. Charles Faiman, Department of Endocrinology, Diabetes, and Metabolism, Cleveland Clinic.)

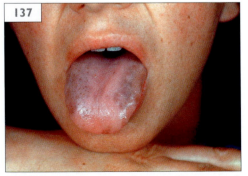

137 Hyperpigmentation of tongue. (Courtesy of Dr. Charles Faiman, Department of Endocrinology, Diabetes, and Metabolism, Cleveland Clinic.)

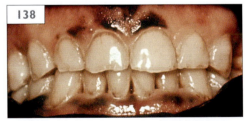

138 Hyperpigmentation of gingival mucosa. (Courtesy of Dr. Charles Faiman, Department of Endocrinology, Diabetes, and Metabolism, Cleveland Clinic.)

Patients may present with a low-grade fever and have varying degrees of gastrointestinal symptoms, which can be confused with acute abdomen with catastrophic consequences.

Secondary adrenal insufficiency presents more insidiously and patients do not manifest skin hyperpigmentation, salt-craving, metabolic acidosis, or hyperkalemia. Fatigue, hyponatremia, and hypoglycemia are the predominant clinical manifestations in secondary adrenal insufficiency.

## DIAGNOSIS

Confirmation of the clinical diagnosis of adrenal insufficiency involves the following three steps (**139**):

- Establishing the presence of adrenal insufficiency.
- Determining the status of ACTH secretion to differentiate primary and secondary causes.
- Investigating the underlying etiology.

**Table 13 Manifestations of primary adrenal insufficiency**

| Symptom | Frequency (%) | Signs | Frequency (%) |
|---|---|---|---|
| Weakness, fatigue | 100 | Weight loss | 100 |
| Anorexia | 100 | Hyperpigmentation | 95 |
| Nausea and/or vomiting | 90 | Hypotension (systolic BP <100 mmHg) | 85–90 |
| Constipation | 20–30 | Vitiligo | 10–15 |
| Diarrhea | 15–20 | **Laboratory abnormalities** | |
| Abdominal pain | 30–35 | Hyponatremia | 80–90 |
| Salt craving | 15–20 | Hyperkalemia | 60–65 |
| Dizziness and/or syncope | 12–15 | Hypercalcemia | 10–20 |
| | | Azotemia | 50–60 |
| | | Anemia and eosinophilia | 20-40 |

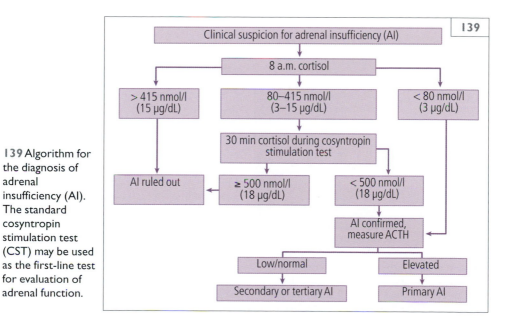

**139** Algorithm for the diagnosis of adrenal insufficiency (AI). The standard cosyntropin stimulation test (CST) may be used as the first-line test for evaluation of adrenal function.

### Establishing the presence of adrenal insufficiency

#### Morning serum cortisol

In normal subjects, serum cortisol concentrations are highest about 1 hr before awakening ranging from 275 to 550 nmol/L (10–20 µg/dL). An early morning cortisol level <80 nmol/l (3 µg/dL) is consistent with adrenal insufficiency, while a value > 415 nmol/L (15 µg/dL) makes the diagnosis highly unlikely. Cortisol levels in the range between 80 and 415 nmol/L (3–15 µg/dL) may be seen in patients with primary or secondary adrenal insufficiency. Such patients should be further evaluated by ACTH stimulation test (cosyntropin stimulation test, CST). Due to the diurnal variation of cortisol, random serum cortisol levels are only of value during stress.

#### Cosyntropin stimulation test

During the standard dose CST, plasma cortisol is measured before, 30, and 60 minutes after an intravenous or intramuscular injection of 250 µg cosyntropin. A normal response is plasma cortisol concentration >500 nmol/L (18 µg/dL) at 30 minutes. The standard dose CST is an excellent test to exclude primary adrenal insufficiency. However, patients with recent onset pituitary ACTH or hypothalamic CRH deficiency (e.g. within 2–4 weeks after pituitary surgery) may have a normal response since adrenal glands have not undergone sufficient atrophy and still respond to very high concentrations of ACTH. The sensitivity of CST to diagnose mild adrenal insufficiency may improve with use of the low-dose CST (1 µg cosyntropin given intravenously); however, this may result in a higher false-positive rate.

#### Other tests

Insulin tolerance test (ITT) and metyrapone test are generally used for the evaluation of patients suspected to have secondary adrenal insufficiency, to evaluate the integrity of the whole hypothalamic–pituitary–adrenal (HPA) axis. ITT is considered the gold standard test for the evaluation of the HPA axis. Metyrapone blocks the final step in cortisol biosynthesis resulting in a reduction in cortisol secretion, which in turn stimulates ACTH secretion leading to a rise in 11-deoxycortisol.

### Differentiation between primary and secondary adrenal insufficiency

An elevated ACTH level (usually >22 pmol/L or 100 pg/mL) in a patient with a low serum cortisol level is consistent with primary AI. A low or normal range ACTH in the same setting confirms the diagnosis of secondary AI.

### Investigating the underlying etiology

The diagnosis of autoimmune adrenal insufficiency is made through the exclusion of the other causes and is supported by the presence of other autoimmune disorders and adrenal autoantibodies, which may be present in up to 80–90% of patients and may be detected before the development of overt adrenal dysfunction. The commonly used antibody measurements include nonspecific adrenal cortical antibodies (ACAs) and antisteroid 21-hydroxylase antibodies (21-OHAbs) which are more sensitive indicators of autoimmune adrenal disease.

Abdominal CT scan may be useful in detecting enlarged adrenal glands and plain X-ray of abdomen can sometimes detect adrenal calcifications (**140**), which may suggest infectious, hemorrhagic, or metastatic causes. In patients diagnosed to have autoimmune adrenal insufficiency, the presence of other endocrine gland dysfunction should be sought.

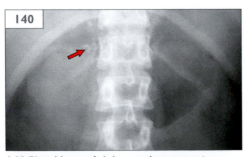

**140** Plain X-ray of abdomen demonstrating adrenal calcification on the right side (arrow) in a patient with a history of adrenal insufficiency secondary to tuberculosis. (Courtesy of Dr. Charles Faiman, Department of Endocrinology, Diabetes, and Metabolism, Cleveland Clinic.)

The presence of X-linked adrenoleuko-dystrophy and adrenomyeloneuropathy should be excluded in young men, particularly in boys less than 15 years old, who have idiopathic adrenal insufficiency without accompanying neurologic symptoms, by measuring plasma very long chain fatty acids. In patients with secondary AI, a thorough evaluation of other pituitary hormones and MRI of the pituitary gland is indicated.

## ADRENAL INSUFFICIENCY IN THE CRITICALLY ILL PATIENT

In critically ill patients, there is stimulation of the HPA axis, decreased corticosteroid-binding globulin (CBG) levels in serum, and increased affinity of glucocorticoid receptors for cortisol, resulting in an increased free cortisol concentration and action at tissue levels. It has been shown that even partial adrenal insufficiency during critical illness can be lethal.

In critically ill patients with normal cortisol binding proteins, a random serum cortisol level <415 nmol/L (15 µg/dL) or a maximum cortisol value <550 nmol/L (20 µg/dL) during CST is suggestive of adrenal insufficiency. However, since more than 90% of measured total cortisol is bound to CBG and albumin, total serum cortisol concentration is falsely decreased in patients with low CBG and significant hypoalbuminemia (<25 g/L). In such a setting, measurement of serum free cortisol is a better indicator of adrenal function. There is a need for establishing the reference range of serum free cortisol for different degrees of severity of illness in critically ill patients. In patients with equivocal biochemical results, a trial of 2–3 days of stress dose glucocorticoids is appropriate as long as such therapy is discontinued in the absence of any significant hemodynamic improvement.

## MANAGEMENT/TREATMENT
### Treatment of adrenal insufficiency
Patients with primary AI require lifelong replacement with both glucocorticoids and mineralocorticoids. The minimum dose to treat symptoms should be used, starting with hydrocortisone 12.5–15 mg in the morning and 2.5–5 mg in the early afternoon to mimic the normal physiologic pattern. Some patients may need another dose of 2.5–5 mg hydrocortisone around 6 p.m. if fatigue continues later in the day.

Patients require fludrocortisone 0.05–0.2 mg for mineralocorticoid replacement. Patients with secondary adrenal insufficiency do not need mineralocorticoid replacement.

During minor illness (e.g. flu or fever greater than 38°C) the hydrocortisone dose should be doubled for 2–3 days. The inability to ingest hydrocortisone tablets warrants parenteral administration. Most patients can be educated to self-administer hydrocortisone 100 mg intra-muscularly and reduce the risk for an emergency room visit. Hydrocortisone 75 mg/day orally (or parenterally if the patient is nil by mouth) provides adequate glucocorticoid coverage for outpatient surgery. Parenteral hydrocortisone 150– 200 mg/day (in 3–4 divided doses) is needed for major surgery with a rapid taper to normal replacement dose during the recovery period. All patients should carry some form of medical alert. Androgen replacement in the form of 25– 50 mg/day of DHEA may improve sexual function and psychological well-being in women with AI.

### Adrenal crisis
Adrenal crisis is a life-threatening condition and refers to the vasomotor collapse associated with infection, stress, or trauma in a patient with adrenal insufficiency. The clinical features include worsening of the initial symptoms of fatigue, anorexia, nausea, vomiting, and abdo-minal pain, followed by sudden deterioration characterized by refractory hypotension leading to death in untreated patients.

Treatment is directed primarily toward the repletion of circulating glucocorticoids and replacement of sodium and water deficits. Glucocorticoid deficiency should be treated by intravenous administration of 100 mg hydro-cortisone. In patients without a history of AI, a blood sample for cortisol should be drawn prior to administration of hydrocortisone. Large volumes (2–3 L) of 0.9 % saline solution may be initially needed to support blood pressure. Hydrocortisone 50 mg every 6–8 hours should be continued until the patient is hemo-dynamically stable and then gradually tapered to physiologic replacement doses according to the patient's clinical picture. Possible precipitating causes should be actively searched for and treated. Mineralocorticoid replacement is generally not needed in patients receiving more than 100 mg hydrocortisone per day.

# Primary aldosteronism

## DEFINITION
Aldosteronism is a syndrome associated with hypersecretion of aldosterone, which is the most potent mineralocorticoid produced by the adrenals. In primary aldosteronism (PA), the cause for the excess aldosterone production resides within the adrenal gland; in secondary aldosteronism, the stimulus is extra-adrenal such as renal vascular disease.

## EPIDEMIOLOGY/ETIOLOGY
PA is twice as common in females than males, and it usually occurs between the ages of 30 and 50 years. Some investigators suggest that up to 10% of unselected patients with hypertension may have PA. The causes of PA are listed in *Table 14*.

Aldosterone-producing adenoma (APA) is the cause of PA in about 65% of cases. These are usually small (<2 cm in diameter), benign tumors, and have a golden yellow color on their cut surface (**141, 142**). Idiopathic hyperaldosteronism (IHA) may be associated with bilateral micronodular or macronodular adrenal hyperplasia and is the second most common cause of PA. Unilateral adrenal hyperplasia and adrenocortical carcinoma are rare causes of PA. Glucocorticoid-remediable aldosteronism (GRA or familial hyperaldosteronism type I) is inherited as an autosomal dominant trait and occurs in childhood or young adulthood. GRA has not been described in African Americans.

## PATHOPHYSIOLOGY
The secretion of aldosterone from the zona glomerulosa is regulated through the renin–angiotensin system, potassium concentration and, to a minor degree, by ACTH. Hypersecretion of aldosterone increases the renal distal tubular exchange of intratubular sodium for potassium and hydrogen ions, leading to hypokalemia and metabolic alkalosis. The excessive sodium reabsorption leads to hypervolemia and low plasma renin level.

GRA results from the expression of a chimeric gene comprising the genetic elements that encode two closely related steroidogenic enzymes, 11β-hydroxylase (CYP11B1) and aldosterone synthase (CYP11B2). In this condition, the aldosterone secretion from the zona fasciculata is regulated primarily by ACTH and not angiotensin II and is suppressible by glucocorticoids.

**Table 14 Causes of primary aldosteronism**
- Aldosterone-producing adenoma (60–65%)
  - including aldosterone-producing renin-responsive adenoma
- Idiopathic hyperaldosteronism (bilateral adrenal hyperplasia) (30–35%)
- Unilateral adrenal hyperplasia (rare)
- Adrenal carcinoma (<5%)
- Familial hyperaldosteronism (FH) (1–3%)
  a. FH- type I (glucocorticoid- remediable aldosteronism)
  b. FH- type II

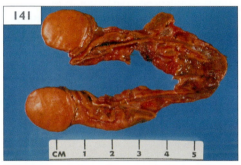

**141** The cut surface of a resected aldosterone-producing adenoma showing a 1.8 cm discrete golden nodule within the cortex of a bivalved adrenal gland. (Courtesy of Dr. Howard Levin, Department of Anatomic Pathology, Cleveland Clinic.)

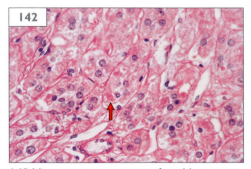

**142** Microscopic appearance of an aldosterone-producing adenoma showing uniform cells with round nuclei and abundant cytoplasm. A spironolactone body is present in the center (arrow). (Courtesy of Dr. Howard Levin, Department of Anatomic Pathology, Cleveland Clinic.)

## CLINICAL PRESENTATION

Patients with PA may be asymptomatic or have symptoms due to hypertension and/or hypokalemia. Patients may have headaches, polyuria, nocturia, polydipsia, paresthesias, weakness, and muscle cramps. There are no specific physical findings. The degree of hypertension is usually moderate to severe, and may be refractory to conventional antihypertensive agents. Malignant hypertension and leg edema are rare. The left ventricular hypertrophy is disproportionate to the level of blood pressure and improves after treatment of hyperaldosteronism even if hypertension persists.

Routine laboratory tests may show mild hypernatremia (143–147 mmol/L), hypokalemia, metabolic alkalosis, and hypomagnesemia. Up to 50% of the patients may have normal potassium concentration. Hypokalemia may occur either spontaneously or after thiazide or loop diuretic use and it may be severe and difficult to correct. Hypokalemia reduces the secretion of aldosterone, and for this reason, serum potassium should be corrected before laboratory evaluation of PA.

GRA should be considered in patients with hypertension in childhood or young adulthood, especially in those with a family history of cardiovascular and cerebrovascular accidents at a young age.

## DIAGNOSIS

PA should be considered in patients with hypertension who develop spontaneous or thiazide-induced hypokalemia, are resistant to therapy, or are diagnosed with an adrenal incidentaloma. The work-up of a patient for PA comprises the following three steps (**143**):
- Screening tests.
- Establishing the autonomy of aldosterone secretion (confirmatory tests).
- Tests to establish the source of aldosterone excess.

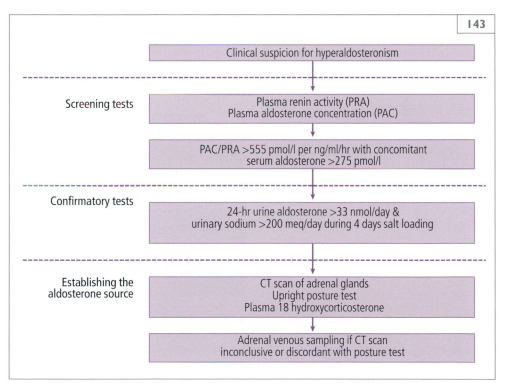

**143** Algorithm for the work-up of patients with suspected primary hyperaldosteronism.

## Screening tests

While hypokalemia in a hypertensive patient is suggestive of PA, normokalemia does not exclude the diagnosis. Adequate sodium intake may be necessary to unmask the hypokalemia. Inappropriate urinary potassium excretion of more than 30 mmol per 24 hr in a patient with hypokalemia suggests PA, especially if plasma renin activity (PRA) is low.

The ratio of plasma aldosterone concentration to the plasma renin activity (PAC/PRA) is the best initial screening test for PA. The test can be done while the patient is on antihypertensive medications (except spirono-lactone and eplerenone) without the need for postural stimulation. Both spironolactone and eplerenone should be discontinued for 6 weeks prior to biochemical testing and potassium should be replaced to the normal range. A PAC (pmol/L)/PRA (ng/mL per hour ) ratio >555 (20, if PAC is expressed as ng/dL) with a concomitant PAC >275 pmol/L (10 ng/dL) needs to be pursued by confirmatory tests (**143**). A low PRA during therapy while on ACE inhibitors or angiotensin receptor blockers (ARB) is suggestive of PA.

## Confirmatory tests

An elevated PAC/PRA by itself is not diagnostic for PA and must be confirmed by measurement of 24-hour urinary aldosterone excretion during 3–5 days of oral salt loading. Diuretics, ACE inhibitors, and ARBs should be discontinued for 2 weeks prior to the test and potassium needs to be replaced to the normal range. A urinary sodium level of more than 200 mmol/24 hours confirms an adequate salt load. An aldosterone excretion of >33 nmol (12 µg)/day during salt loading is almost always diagnostic of PA.

Intravenous administration of 2 liters of isotonic saline over 4 hours in the supine position is a less favored way to establish the diagnosis. Plasma aldosterone >275 pmol/L (10 ng/dL) at the end of the infusion supports the diagnosis of PA. This test may not be safe in elderly patients with uncontrolled hypertension or decompensated heart disease. A lack of decrease in aldosterone level following administration of captopril also supports the diagnosis of PA.

Dexamethasone suppression test is used for the diagnosis of GRA. In patients with hyperaldosteronism, plasma aldosterone level <111 pmol/L (4 ng/dL) in the morning after 2 days of dexamethasone (0.5 mg every 6 hours) is suggestive of GRA. Such patients should be referred for genetic testing for definitive diagnosis.

## Tests to establish the source of aldosterone excess

Because of differences in therapy, distinguishing between APA and IHA is important. Patients with APA generally have more severe hypertension, more frequent hypokalemia, higher plasma and urinary aldosterone levels, and are younger (<50 years old). APA is typically hypodense (<10 Hounsfield units) and <2 cm in size on the CT scan of adrenals (**144**).

Plasma 18-hydroxycorticosterone levels and posture test can be of further help to distinguish APA from IHA. A plasma 18-hydroxycorticosterone level of >2800 nmol/mL (100 ng/dL) supports the diagnosis of APA. During the posture test, PAC is measured before and 2 hours after upright posture (with ambulation). Patients with APA show a <30% increase or a paradoxical decrease in PAC compared to those with IHA.

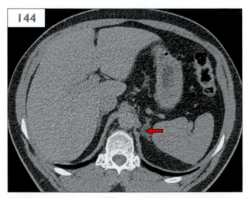

**144** Non-contrast CT scan of adrenal glands in a patient with primary aldosteronism showing a 2 cm nodule in the left adrenal gland with Hounsfield units <10, suggesting a benign adenoma (arrow).

Patients with an adrenal mass >1 cm in one adrenal and the posture test suggestive of APA do not need any further testing and may proceed with surgery. Those without a definite adrenal mass or discordant results should be referred for adrenal venous sampling. The adrenal veins are catheterized by the percutaneous femoral vein approach. Venous sampling of both adrenal veins and the inferior vena cava below the renal veins is performed during continuous ACTH infusion (**145A, B**). The test relies on demonstration of a gradient for plasma aldosterone in unilateral disease. Cortisol should be measured in order to confirm the proper catheter placement in adrenal veins.

## MANAGEMENT/TREATMENT

The treatment goal is to reduce morbidity and mortality including cardiovascular damage associated with hypertension, hypokalemia, and hyperaldosteronism by normalization of blood pressure and aldosterone levels. Unilateral adrenalectomy by a laparoscopic approach results in normalization of hypokalemia and resolution or improvement in hypertension. About half of the patients become normotensive without drug therapy. The blood pressure response to spironolactone before surgery often predicts the blood pressure response to the surgery in those with APA.

Medical treatment is reserved for patients with IHA or those with APA who are poor surgical candidates. Spironolactone in a dose of 50–200 mg per day is the treatment of choice. The side-effects include painful gynecomastia, nausea, headaches, impotence, and irregular menstruation. Serum potassium and magnesium should be monitored to avoid hyperkalemia and hypomagnesemia. Eplerenone is a more selective aldosterone receptor antagonist and has a better side-effect profile, but is less potent compared to spironolactone.

In patients with GRA, hypertension is usually controlled by treatment with glucocorticoids in low doses (0.125–0.5 mg of dexamethasone or 2.5–5 mg of prednisone per day). Complete suppression of ACTH-regulated aldosterone production is not usually necessary and raises the risk of development of cushingoid features. Spironolactone and amiloride are alternative treatments. Genetic counseling is advisable for patients with this autosomal dominant disorder.

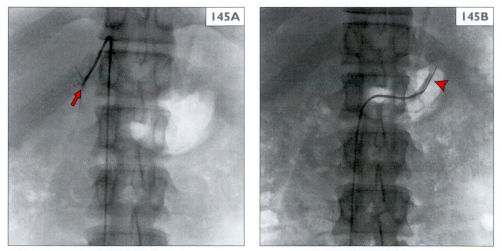

**145** Abdominal radiographs which shows adrenal venous sampling for identifying the source of hyperaldosteronism. Catheter is placed in the right adrenal (**A**; arrow) and the left adrenal (**B**; arrowhead).

# Pheochromocytoma

### DEFINITION

Pheochromocytomas are catecholamine-producing neuroendocrine tumors arising from chromaffin cells of the adrenal medulla or extra-adrenal paraganglia (paragangliomas).

### ANATOMY/ETIOLOGY

Most pheochromocytomas are benign, sporadic, unilateral, and located within the adrenal gland (**146, 147**). Extra-adrenal pheochromocytomas (paragangliomas) occur in about 15% of cases: superior and inferior para-aortic areas including organ of Zuckerkandl (75%), the bladder (10%), thorax (10%), head, neck, and pelvis (5%). Paragangliomas tend to occur in younger patients (<20 years) and are uncommon in those older than age 60. Bilateral adrenal pheochromocytomas (5–10% of cases) usually occur as part of the familial syndromes. Although metastases might be rare for adrenal pheochromocytomas (5–10%), the prevalence of malignant disease is about 33% for extra-adrenal pheochromocytomas. Tumors >5 cm in size have a greater potential to metastasize.

Familial predisposition to pheochromocytoma is seen in patients with multiple endocrine neoplasia (MEN) types 2A and 2B, Von Hippel–Lindau (VHL) disease, neurofibromatosis type 1 (NF-1), and familial pheochromocytoma/paraganglioma syndromes. Genetic screening in patients with apparently sporadic pheochromocytoma is recommended for those with paragangliomas, bilateral disease, and age under 20 years.

MEN2A is characterized by MTC, pheochromocytoma, and primary parathyroid hyperplasia, whereas MEN2B includes MTC, pheochromocytoma, mucosal neuromas, and a marfanoid body habitus, but not hyperparathyroidism. Mutations in the *RET*

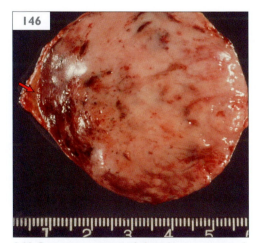

146 Gross appearance of pheochromocytoma. A 6 cm predominantly gray-tan mass with some areas of hemorrhage is seen within the substance of the adrenal gland. A small remnant of normal adrenal cortex is visible (arrow). (Courtesy of Dr. Howard Levin, Department of Anatomic Pathology, Cleveland Clinic.)

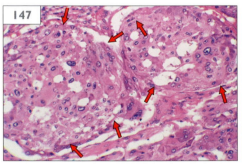

147 Microscopic appearance of pheochromocytoma. Cell balls ('zellballen') (arrows) are demarcated by connective tissue containing capillaries. Nuclei are round to oval. Cytoplasm is pink, somewhat granular, and focally vacuolated. (Courtesy of Dr. Howard Levin, Department of Anatomic Pathology, Cleveland Clinic.)

proto-oncogene in chromosome 10, which codes for a tyrosine kinase receptor, have been implicated in over 90% of families with MEN2. Pheochromocytoma is the first clinical manifestation in 10–30% of patients with MEN2. Most patients (50–80%) develop bilateral adrenal tumors. Extra-adrenal tumors and malignant disease are uncommon (<5%).

## CLINICAL FEATURES

Hypertension is the most common clinical manifestation of pheochromocytoma and is present in more than 90% of the patients. Wide fluctuations in blood pressure and resistance to antihypertensive medications are typical of pheochromocytoma. The triad of headaches, palpitations, and diaphoresis suggests the diagnosis; however, the absence of these symptoms does not exclude the disease. Attacks are usually precipitated by emotional stress, exercise, anesthesia, abdominal pressure, or ingestion of tyramine-containing foods. Both pallor and flushing may be seen in patients. Other symptoms include orthostatic hypotension, weight loss, dyspnea, polyuria, polydipsia, visual blurring, focal neurologic symptoms, change in mental status, myocardial infarction, heart failure, hypertensive encephalopathy, CVA, and pulmonary edema.

## DIAGNOSIS

The indications for screening of patients suspected to have pheochromocytoma are listed in *Table 15*. The measurement of plasma metanephrines (metanephrine and normeta-nephrine) or 24-hour urine metanephrines is a reasonable first-line screening test for pheochromocytoma.

Plasma metanephrines have a higher sensitivity (97–99%) than other biochemical tests for diagnosis of both sporadic and familial pheochromocytoma. However, it is associated with a false-positive rate of 10–15%. In general, plasma metanephrines more than 3–4 times the upper limit of normal for the assay is diagnostic of pheochromocytoma. Patients with

---

**Table 15 Indications for screening of patients suspected to have pheochromocytoma**

- Episodic symptoms of headaches, tachycardia, and diaphoresis (with or without hypertension)

- Family history of pheochromocytoma or familial syndromes that may include pheochromocytoma

- Adrenal incidentaloma

- Unexplained paroxysms of tachy-/bradyarrhythmias or hypertension during induction of anesthesia, surgery, or parturition or prolonged and unexplained postoperative hypotension

- Adverse cardiovascular reactions to certain drugs including anesthetic agents, beta-blockers, glucagon, tricyclic antidepressants, histamine, phenothiazine, and tyramine-containing foods

- Spells or attacks during exertion, movements of torso, straining, coitus, or micturition

- Refractory or labile hypertension

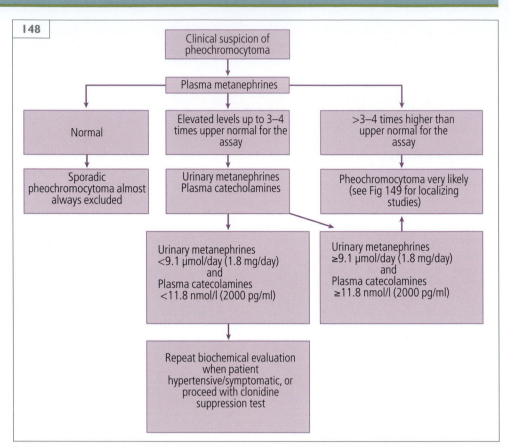

**148** Algorithm for the biochemical evaluation of patients suspected to have pheochromocytoma.

**Table 16  List of medications and stimulants to avoid before the measurement of plasma and urinary catecholamines and metanephrines**

Tricyclic antidepressants

Beta-blockers: labetalol* and sotalol

Acetaminophen

Phenoxybenzamine

Monoamine oxidase inhibitors

Antipsychotics

Sympathomimetics: ephedrine, pseudoephedrine, amphetamines, albuterol

Stimulants: caffeine, nicotine, theophylline

Miscellaneous: levodopa, carbidopa, alcohol, cocaine

*Labetalol interferes only with certain assays

intermediate levels of plasma metanephrines should have their urinary metanephrines measured, or undergo clonidine suppression test if hypertensive (**148**). Patients should avoid caffeinated beverages and alcohol for 24 hours and the medications listed in *Table 16* for 3–5 days (2 weeks for labetalol in certain assays) prior to biochemical evaluation.

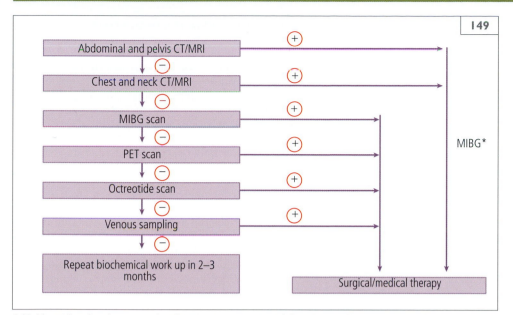

149 Algorithm for the tumor localization in patients with biochemically proven pheochromocytoma (PHEO). MIBG: [123]I-metaiodobenzylguanidine; PET: positron emission tomography.
*In patients with positive finding on CT/MRI imaging, MIBG scan may be considered in those with familial PHEO, young age (<20 yr), ectopic PHEO, and tumors larger than 5 cm in size.

## Imaging studies

Pheochromocytomas are usually >3 cm in diameter and tend to be cystic with areas of necrosis. In patients suspected to have a pheochromocytoma, noncontrast CT scan of abdomen and pelvis should be performed, followed by CT scan of chest and neck if no tumor is found (**149**). CT scan has a sensitivity of 93–100% for detecting adrenal pheochromocytoma and approximately 90% for extra-adrenal pheochromocytomas (**150**). An adrenal tumor with a maximum noncontrast CT Hounsfield unit <10 is extremely unlikely to be a pheochromocytoma.

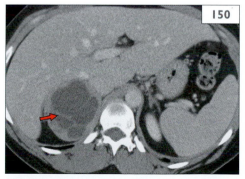

150 Pheochromocytoma: CT scan of adrenal glands showing an 8 cm right adrenal mass, with central necrosis (arrow). The mass deforms the contour of the liver without evidence of invasion.

MRI has a similar sensitivity compared to CT scan for detecting adrenal pheochromocytomas but is superior for detecting extra-adrenal tumors. Pheochromocytomas exhibit signal isointensity with liver, kidney, and muscle on T1 and a characteristic high signal intensity on T2-weighted images (**151**).

Functional imaging using $^{123}$I-metaiodobenzylguanidine (MIBG) offers superior specificity (95–100%) and is helpful in diagnosing extra-adrenal pheochromocytoma and metastasis (**152A, B**). However, a negative examination does not exclude pheochromocytoma (sensitivity 77–90%). Some of the indications for obtaining MIBG scan include: lack of tumor localization by conventional imaging methods in patients with positive biochemical results, younger than age 20, familial pheochromocytoma, tumor >5 cm in size, and extra-adrenal location.

Positron emission tomography (PET) with $^{18}$F-fluorodopamine, $^{18}$F-fluorodopa, or $^{18}$F-fluorodeoxyglucose (FDG) and somatostatin receptor imaging using $^{111}$Indium- labeled octreotide (Octreoscan) are other functional imaging methods that may be used if MIBG scanning is negative.

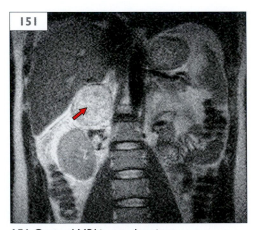

**151** Coronal MRI image showing a heterogeneous 6 cm right adrenal mass exhibiting a bright T2 signal intensity suggestive of pheochromocytoma (arrow).

## DIFFERENTIAL DIAGNOSIS

Abrupt withdrawal from medications such as clonidine or from alcohol may mimic the symptoms of pheochromocytoma and cause elevations in catecholamines. Conditions such as pre-eclampsia, subarachnoid hemorrhage, and migraine may mimic pheochromocytoma. Agents such as amphetamines, ephedrine, pseudoephedrine, isoproterenol, cocaine, phencyclidine, and lysergic acid diethylamide may also lead to excess catecholamine levels.

On the other hand, the symptoms of pheochromocytoma may be mistaken for those of panic attacks, hypoglycemic episodes, or accelerated hypertension of other etiologies. Lastly, disorders such as mastocytosis and the carcinoid syndrome, which are characterized by spells and episodic symptoms, may also mimic pheochromocytoma. However, hypertensive crises, which often occur with pheochromocytoma, are very rare in these disorders.

## MANAGEMENT/TREATMENT
### Preoperative management

The definitive treatment for pheochromocytoma is surgical excision of the tumor. Adequate medical preparation is essential and is usually achieved in 10–14 days. Alpha-adrenoceptor blockers and dihydropyridine calcium channel blockers are the commonly used agents. The first-line agents are doxazosin (selective postsynaptic $\alpha_1$-blocker) and phenoxybenzamine (long-acting, noncompetitive α-blocker). The use of phenoxybenzamine is associated with more side-effects and could result in prolonged postoperative hypotension. A β-adrenoceptor blocker (e.g. propranolol or atenolol) could be added after initiation of α-adrenergic blockade in patients who are tachycardic. Blockade of β-adrenoceptors should never be initiated before α-adrenoceptor blockade, since the unopposed α-adrenoceptor stimulation may result in hypertensive crises. Calcium channel blockers could be used for surgical preparation or may be added to the antihypertensive regimen if there is persistent or episodic hypertension. Acute hypertensive crises can be treated with intravenous nitroprusside, nitroglycerine, short-acting alpha-blocker, phentolamine, magnesium sulphate, and calcium channel blocker, nicardipine.

## Surgical management

Surgery for pheochromocytoma has shifted from the open conventional to laparoscopic approach over the past decade. A laparoscopic procedure reduces postoperative morbidity, hospital stay, and expense compared to conventional laparotomy. Close blood pressure monitoring by an experienced anesthesiologist is necessary during surgery. Antihypertensive agents need to be withheld postoperatively with close monitoring of blood pressure and blood glucose levels. Long-term follow-up is necessary in all patients.

Malignant pheochromocytomas are diagnosed by the presence of extra-adrenal metastases, commonly in the bones, lungs, liver, and lymph nodes. Metastases should be resected if possible. Alternatives to surgical resection include external beam radiation, cryoablation, radiofrequency ablation, trans-catheter arterial embolization, chemotherapy, and radiopharmaceutical therapy.

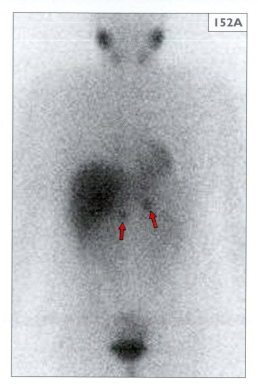

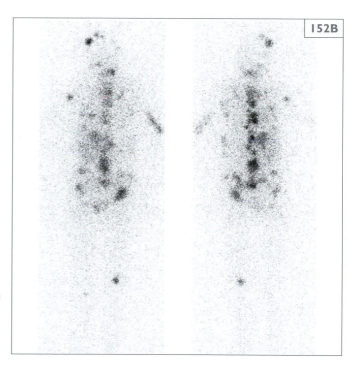

**152** $^{123}$I-metaiodo-benzylguanidine (MIBG) scan of patients with bilateral pheochromocytoma (**A**) and metastatic pheochromo-cytoma (**B**). Arrows indicate abnormal uptake in the region of adrenals in (A). (Courtesy of Dr. Donald Neumann, Department of Nuclear Medicine, Cleveland Clinic.)

# Cushing syndrome

### DEFINITION
Cushing syndrome (CS) comprises the symptoms and signs associated with prolonged exposure to inappropriately elevated levels of free plasma glucocorticoids.

### ETIOLOGY/PATHOPHYSIOLOGY
The etiology of CS can be classified into ACTH-dependent and ACTH-independent. If CS due to exogenous glucocorticoids is excluded, primary ACTH-independent adrenal etiologies account for 15–20% of endogenous CS in adults, of which approximately 90% are unilateral tumors (*Table 17*). Benign adenomas represent up to 80% of these cases (**153**). Adrenal etiologies account for 65% of CS in prepubertal children.

Adrenal tumors are more frequent in females than males, with a ratio of 4:1 for adenomas and 2:1 for adrenocortical carcinomas. Adrenocortical carcinomas are 3–4 times more likely to be the cause of CS in children.

Bilateral macronodular adrenal hyperplasia (BMAH) is a rare cause of CS and is estimated to represent less than 1% of endogenous cases (**154, 155**). It should not be confused with the more common bilateral adrenal hyperplasia in ACTH-dependent CS due to chronic stimulation of adrenal glands by ACTH (**156, 157**). In CS due to McCune–Albright syndrome, activating mutations of $G_{s\alpha}$ receptor in adrenal cells lead to formation of adrenal nodules in which constitutive activation of the cyclic AMP pathway leads to excess cortisol secretion.

**Table 17  Causes of adrenal Cushing syndrome**

**Unilateral**

Benign adrenal adenoma

Adrenocortical carcinoma

Unilateral adrenocortical hyperplasia

**Bilateral**

Bilateral macronodular hyperplasia

Primary pigmented nodular adrenocortical disease and Carney's complex

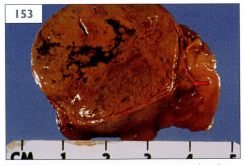

**153** Adrenal cortical adenoma associated with Cushing syndrome: a well encapsulated 3.6 cm yellow-tan intra-adrenal mass with focal hemorrhage. Normal adrenal tissue is seen to the right (arrow). (Courtesy of Dr. Howard Levin, Department of Anatomic Pathology, Cleveland Clinic.)

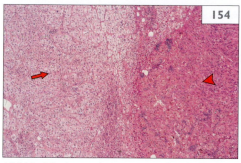

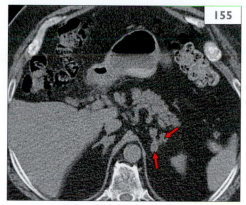

**154** Nodular hyperplasia associated with Cushing syndrome: coalescing large nodules are seen, which are comprised of cells with clear cytoplasm (arrow) and eosinophilic cytoplasm (arrowhead). (Courtesy of Dr. Howard Levin, Department of Anatomic Pathology, Cleveland Clinic.)

**155** Noncontrast CT scan of abdomen in a patient with bilateral macronodular adrenal hyperplasia showing bilateral 1–2 cm nodules in the adrenals (arrows).

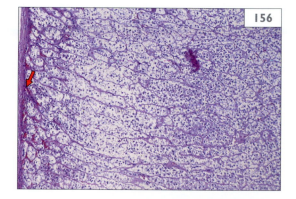

**156** Diffuse cortical hyperplasia in a patient with pituitary Cushing syndrome. There is marked expansion of the zona fasciculata and reticularis. The zona glomerulosa is not visible. The normal capsule is seen to the left (arrow). (Courtesy of Dr. Howard Levin, Department of Anatomic Pathology, Cleveland Clinic.)

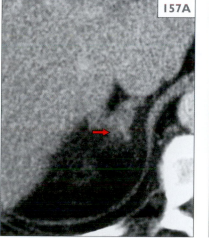

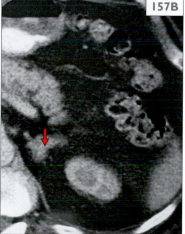

**157** CT scan of abdomen in a patient with pituitary Cushing syndrome showing bilateral enlarged adrenal glands (arrows). The adrenals tend to maintain their shape.

## Primary pigmented nodular adrenocortical disease and Carney's complex

Primary pigmented nodular adrenocortical disease (PPNAD) is caused by autonomously functioning bilateral small pigmented adrenal nodules (**158A, B**). Patients are usually younger than age 30 and there is a positive family history in about 50% of the cases. The familial PPNAD is called Carney complex and may include blue nevi, atrial myxomas, spotty skin pigmentation, peripheral nerve tumors, and various tumors including breast, testicular, and growth hormone-secreting pituitary adenomas. Inactivating mutations of the type 1a regulatory subunit of cyclic AMP-dependent protein kinase A gene has been observed in a higher proportion of PPNAD patients.

## Aberrant hormone receptors in adrenal CS

Recent evidence shows that cortisol production by some adrenal tumors are triggered or promoted by aberrant expression and pathologic activation of several G-protein coupled receptors, such as those of vasopressin, gastric inhibitory peptide (GIP), vasoactive intestinal polypeptide (VIP), LH/hCG, and catecholamines. Different stimuli such as posture, food, and pregnancy may result in excessive release of cortisol from the adrenal tumor, resulting in clinical manifestations of CS.

## CLINICAL PRESENTATION

Some of the clinical features suggestive of CS are listed in *Table 18*. Among these, skin manifestations and serial photographs warrant special attention (**159**). The striae in CS are

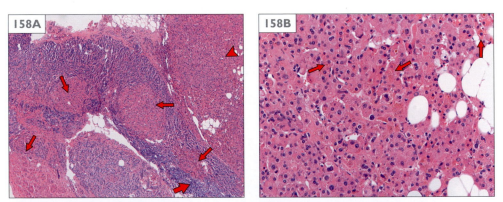

**158** Primary pigmented nodular adrenocortical disease. In low power magnification (**A**), four discrete intracortical eosinophilic nodules are seen (arrows). **A** larger nodule extends into periadrenal fat (arrowhead). A strip of normal medullary tissue is present in the lower center right (large arrow). **B**: High-power magnification of an eosinophilic nodule present within periadrenal fat. There is mild variation in nuclear size. Many adrenal cortical cells contain abundant fine brown lipochrome pigment (arrows), accounting for the black color of nodules in gross specimen. (Courtesy of Dr. Howard Levin, Department of Anatomic Pathology, Cleveland Clinic.)

**Table 18 Clinical features suggestive of Cushing syndrome**

- Central obesity
- Proximal myopathy
- Spontaneous bruising
- Facial plethora

- Wide purplish striae (>1 cm)
- Changes in serial photographs
- Hypokalemia
- Osteoporosis

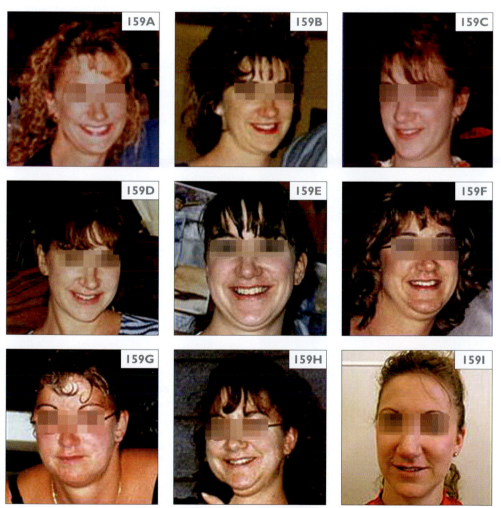

**159** Serial photographs of a patient with Cushing syndrome demonstrating gradual development of moon face, acne, and facial plethora. The patient underwent surgery in 2003. Note the dramatic improvement in the facial appearance 9 months after surgery. **A** = 1995; **B** = 1996; **C** = 1998; **D** = 1999; **E** = 2000; **F** = 2001; **G** = 2002; **H** = 2003; **I** = 2004. (Not taken as clinical pictures)

red-purple in color and usually greater than 1 cm in width (**160A, B**). Skin is thinned, wrinkled (Liddle's sign – 'cigarette paper' on the dorsum of the hands) and minimal trauma results in easy bruising. Face has a plethoric appearance and acne may be present. Patients may have myopathy involving the proximal muscles of the lower limb and the shoulder girdle. Supraclavicular and dorsocervical fat pads (buffalo hump) are nonspecific findings and may be seen in most patients presenting to obesity clinics. Both sexes complain of decreased libido and women may present with irregular menstruation and hirsutism.

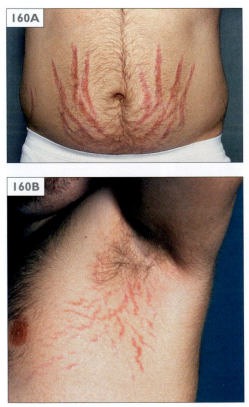

**160** Abdominal (**A**) and axillary striae (**B**) in a patient with Cushing syndrome. The striae are purple and broad (>1cm in width). (Courtesy of Dr. Charles Faiman, Department of Endocrinology, Diabetes, and Metabolism, Cleveland Clinic.)

Hypertension and hypokalemia may be seen in patients with CS and are mainly due to the binding of excess cortisol to the nonspecific type 1 aldosterone receptors. Virilization may be a part of the clinical picture in patients with adrenocortical carcinoma cosecreting androgens. The onset of clinical features is usually gradual in patients with adrenal adenomas but often rapid in adrenocortical carcinomas.

Some of the patients (5–20%) with incidentally detected adrenal masses (adrenal incidentalomas) have evidence of mild cortisol hypersecretion in the absence of the typical clinical features of CS. Such patients develop clinical manifestations of adrenal insufficiency following removal of the adrenal tumor due to chronic suppression of contralateral adrenal gland. This has been termed subclinical CS (SCS). There is some evidence of increased incidence of cardiovascular risk factors such as obesity, hypertension, hyperlipidemia, and hyperinsulinemia in patients with SCS, but long-term studies are lacking.

### DIAGNOSIS

Once CS due to exogenous administration of glucocorticoids is excluded, the evaluation of a patient with suspected CS should take place in two stages: (1) establishing hypercortisolemia (confirm presence of CS), and (2) establishing the etiology of CS (**161**).

The diagnosis of CS has been dealt with in detail in Chapter 4 Hypothalamic–pituitary disorders. Serum ACTH level should be measured once hypercortisolemia is established. ACTH concentrations below 2.2 pmol/L (10 pg/mL) are consistent with an ACTH-independent CS secondary to an adrenal etiology. Once the diagnosis of ACTH-independent CS has been established, the adrenals need to be imaged by noncontrast CT scan. In patients with unilateral hyperfunctioning adrenal tumor, the contralateral adrenal gland is usually atrophic. MRI has a similar diagnostic value as CT in differentiating benign and malignant adrenal masses. However, in patients with suspected adrenocortical carcinoma, MRI provides more information about vascular invasion, particularly the inferior vena cava and the adrenal and renal veins.

In BMAH, the adrenal glands can be replaced by the presence of numerous nodules up to 4 cm in diameter (see **155**); in other cases, the adrenal appears diffusely enlarged without macroscopic nodules. In PPNAD, imaging of the adrenal glands may reveal slightly enlarged glands with or without discernible nodules. The clinical diagnosis of virilization secondary to an adrenal tumor may be confirmed by the measurements of serum DHEAS and testosterone and 24-hour urinary excretion of 17-ketosteroids. Feminization can be confirmed by the measurement of elevated plasma levels of estradiol and/or estrone.

## DIFFERENTIAL DIAGNOSIS

A pseudo-Cushing's state can be defined as some or all of the clinical features of CS together with some evidence for hypercortisolism. Several causes have been described including alcoholism, sleep apnea, depression, obesity, uncontrolled type 2 diabetes, and anorexia nervosa. Resolution of the underlying cause results in disappearance of the cushingoid state.

## MANAGEMENT/TREATMENT

Goals of treatment of CS include normalization of cortisol levels, eradication of the tumor, and avoidance of permanent hormonal deficiency.

Hormone-secreting adrenal adenomas should be surgically removed. Compared to the open adrenalectomy, the laparoscopic approach is associated with decreased postoperative pain, reduced time to return of bowel function, and decreased length of hospital stay. Surgical resection of the adrenocortical carcinoma at an early stage is the only therapy that may offer potential for cure. Bilateral adrenalectomy is recommended for patients with PPNAD and BMAH.

Medical therapy with agents such as ketoconazole, metyrapone, and mitotane may be used in patients who are not surgical candidates and those who could not have a complete tumor resection.

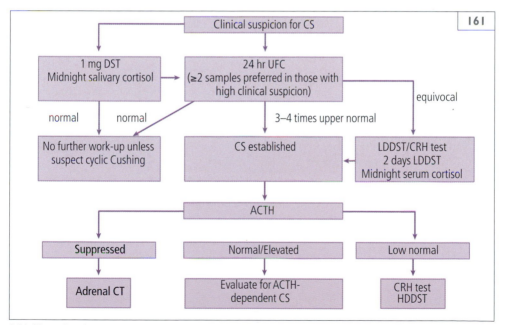

**161** Algorithm for evaluation of patients suspected to have Cushing syndrome. ACTH: adrenocorticotrophic hormone; CRH: corticotrophin-releasing hormone; CS: Cushing syndrome; CT: computed tomography; DST: dexamethasone suppression test; HDDST: high-dose dexamethasone suppression test; LDDST: low-dose dexamethasone suppression test; UFC: urine free cortisol.

# Congenital adrenal hyperplasia

## DEFINITION
Congenital adrenal hyperplasia (CAH) encompasses a group of disorders of adrenal steroid biosynthesis, which are inherited in an autosomal recessive fashion.

## EPIDEMIOLOGY/ETIOLOGY
21-hydroxylase deficiency is the most common cause of CAH, which accounts for at least 90% of all diagnosed cases. Its prevalence based upon neonatal screening studies is about 1 in 14 200 live births, but can be as high as 1/280 in Alaskan Eskimos. Among whites, the prevalence of the mild nonclassic form of the disorder may be as high as 1 in 1000, with the prevalence being higher among Hispanics, Yugoslavs, and Eastern European Jews. The disorder occurs in about 1–2% of white women with clinical evidence of hyperandrogenism. 11β-hydroxylase deficiency is the second most common cause of CAH, with an incidence of 1 in 100 000 live births, and it accounts for about 5–8% of cases of CAH. Other enzyme deficiencies like 3β-hydroxysteroid dehydrogenase deficiency, 17α-hydroxylase deficiency and steroidogenic acute regulatory protein (StAR) protein deficiency are very rare.

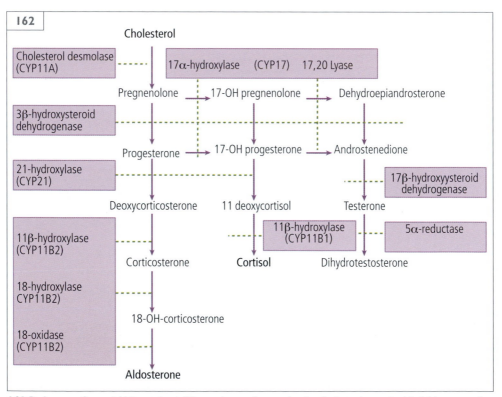

**162** Pathways of steroid biosynthesis. The pathways for synthesis of mineralocorticoids (aldosterone), glucocorticoids (cortisol), and androgens (testosterone and dihydrotestosterone) are arranged from left to right. The enzymes coded by a single gene catalyzing each bioconversion are shown in boxes.

## PATHOGENESIS

Deficient cortisol production is the key aberration in all forms of CAH. 21-hydroxylase (CYP21A2) is a cytochrome P450 enzyme located in the endoplasmic reticulum. It catalyzes the conversion of 17α-hydroxyprogesterone (17-OHP) to 11-deoxycortisol, a precursor of cortisol, and the conversion of progesterone to deoxycorticosterone, a precursor of aldosterone (**162**). CAH due to 21-hydroxylase deficiency is caused by homozygous or compound heterozygous mutations in the human CYP21A2 gene located in the short arm of chromosome 6. As a result there is defective conversion of 17α-hydroxyprogesterone to 11-deoxycortisol and subsequently cortisol. Reduced cortisol biosynthesis results in increased ACTH secretion,

which in turn shunts excess precursors such as 17-hydroxypregnenolone and 17α-hydroxyprogesterone into the pathway for androgen biosynthesis (**163**). Mutations associated with milder reduction in the enzyme activity result in less severe abnormalities and the nonclassic CAH.

## CLINICAL PRESENTATION

The classic CAH due to 21-hydroxylase deficiency is associated with aldosterone deficiency in 75% of patients (salt wasters), which may lead to failure to thrive, hypovolemia, and shock. The rest (25%) produce sufficient aldosterone to prevent salt wasting but present with virilization in genetic females (simple virilizers) and develop glucocorticoid insufficiency at or within a few

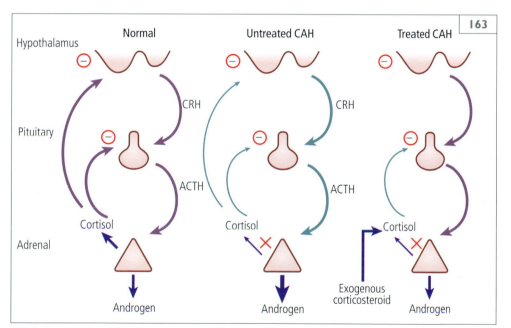

163 Pathogenesis of CAH. In a patient with normal adrenal function, the adrenals produce both cortisol and androgens, and the HPA axis is controlled by negative feedback. In the untreated patient with CAH, the block in cortisol synthesis leads to lack of negative feedback and increased secretion of CRH and ACTH, leading to adrenal hyperplasia and oversecretion of androgens. In the patient with treated CAH, the exogenous corticosteroid replacement leads to suppression of excess androgen secretion.

weeks after birth (**164**). Patients who are inadequately treated show rapid somatic growth and advanced skeletal age, which leads to premature epiphyseal fusion and subsequent short stature. Boys show only subtle hyperpigmentation and penile enlargement. Affected males might develop testicular adrenal rests, which can masquerade as testicular tumors. Newborn females with nonclassic CAH have normal female genitalia. Overproduction of adrenal androgens in adult females results in hirsutism as the most common presenting symptom, followed by oligomenorrhea or amenorrhea, acne, and infertility, closely resembling the polycystic ovarian syndrome (PCOS) (**165A, B**). Male patients may present with acne, short stature, oligospermia, and diminished fertility.

### DIAGNOSIS

Classic 21-hydroxylase deficiency is characterized by markedly elevated serum levels of 17-OHP, which is the main substrate for the enzyme (**162**). Basal 17-OHP values usually exceed 300 nmol/L (10 000 ng/dL) in affected infants, whereas the levels in normal newborns are below 3 nmol/L (100 ng/dL). Levels of DHEAS,

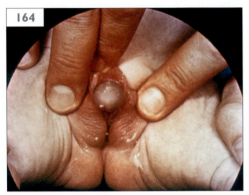

**164** Female infant with classic 21-hydroxylase deficiency presenting with ambiguous genitalia as a result of in utero exposure to excess androgens. (Courtesy of Dr. Charles Faiman, Department of Endocrinology, Diabetes, and Metabolism, Cleveland Clinic.)

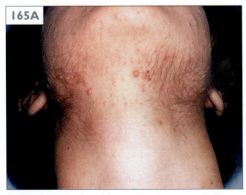

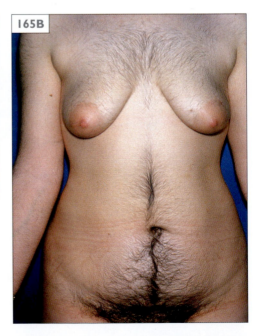

**165** Adult female with nonclassic congenital adrenal hyperplasia presenting with acne, facial (**A**), and body hirsuitism (**B**). (Courtesy of Dr. Charles Faiman, Department of Endocrinology, Diabetes, and Metabolism, Cleveland Clinic.)

testosterone, and androstenedione are increased because of shunting of precursors through the androgen pathway, but are of limited usefulness in the newborn period. PRA is increased in the salt-wasting variety. The diagnosis is confirmed using the ACTH (cosyntropin) stimulation test by measuring 17-OHP at baseline and 60 minutes after injection of 250 µg of cosyntropin. Patients with the salt-wasting disease have the highest 17-OHP levels of up to 3000 nmol/L (100 000 ng/dL) after cosyntropin stimulation, followed by patients with simple virilizing disease, who usually have levels between 300 and 1000 nmol/L (10 000–30 000 ng/dL).

Adults with the nonclassic CAH might have normal or borderline basal 17-OHP. A basal 17-OHP drawn at 8AM in follicular phase of menstrual cycle <6 nmol/L (200 ng/dL) essentially rules out CAH. A 17-OHP value >45 nmol/L (1500 ng/dL) 60 minutes after injection of 250 µg of cosyntropin supports the diagnosis.

## GENETICS
The diagnosis of CAH can be confirmed by genotyping and is part of newborn screening programs in some countries. Mutations in the CYP21 (CYP21A2) gene, which is located in the HLA histocompatibility complex on chromosome 6p21.3 along with a pseudogene, CYP21P (CYP21A1P), are responsible for causing 21-hydroxylase deficiency. There is some correlation between the genotype and the phenotype in CAH patients, and CYP21 mutations can be grouped into three categories based on the enzymatic activity predicted from *in vitro* studies. The first group consists of mutations such as deletions or nonsense mutations that totally ablate enzyme activity; these are most often associated with salt-wasting disease. The second group of mutations yields enzymes with 1–2% of normal activity and these mutations permit adequate aldosterone synthesis and thus are found in patients with simple virilizing disease. The final group includes mutations that produce enzymes retaining 20–60% of normal activity; these mutations are associated with the nonclassic disorder. 11β-hydroxylase deficiency is caused by mutations of the CYP11B1 gene located on chromosome 8q21-q22, where as 17α-hydroxylase deficiency is caused by mutations in CYP17 gene, which is located on chromosome 10.

## DIFFERENTIAL DIAGNOSIS
The major differential diagnosis in adults with nonclassic CAH is PCOS. Clinical symptoms and signs of both these disorders overlap, and the diagnosis is usually established using the ACTH stimulation test and, if indicated, genotyping. Other differential diagnoses include virilizing adrenal and ovarian tumors.

## MANAGEMENT/TREATMENT
The goal of treatment of patients with CAH is adequate suppression of adrenal androgen production without causing cushingoid features. In children, the preferred drug is hydrocortisone in doses of 10–20 mg/m² of body surface area per day in three divided doses. The patient's clinical status, bone age, growth velocity, and Tanner stage, along with the measurement of 17-OHP, DHEAS, testosterone, and androstenedione may be used to adjust the dose. Older adolescents and adults may be treated with prednisone (5–7.5 mg daily in two divided doses) or dexamethasone (total of 0.25–0.5 mg given in one or two doses per day) with careful monitoring to prevent iatrogenic Cushing syndrome. Patients with the salt-wasting form of CAH require supplemental mineralocorticoids (0.05–0.2 mg of fludrocortisone daily). The dose of glucocorticoids needs to be increased during acute illness or stress to prevent adrenal crisis. Patients with ambiguous genitalia should undergo correctional surgery between 2 and 6 months of age.

In pregnancies where the fetus is at risk for classic CAH, maternal dexamethasone treatment instituted early in the first trimester can successfully suppress the fetal HPA axis and prevent the genital ambiguity of affected female infants. Chorionic villus sampling or amniocentesis should be performed for determination of fetal sex and genotyping for the CYP21A2 gene. The treatment with dexamethasone can be safely discontinued if the fetus is male or the female is unaffected.

# Adrenocortical carcinoma

## INCIDENCE/EPIDEMIOLOGY

Adrenocortical carcinomas (ACCs) account for 0.05–0.2% of all cancers, with an approximate prevalence of 2 new cases per 1 million population per year. A bimodal age distribution has been reported, with the first peak occurring before the age 5 and the second in the 4th to 5th decade. Females account for 65–90% of the reported cases. The prevalence of adrenal carcinoma among all incidentally detected adrenal masses is about 1 in 1500.

## MOLECULAR PATHOGENESIS

The molecular pathogenesis of ACC is poorly understood. Long-term observational studies suggest that ACC do not originate from pre-existing adrenal adenomas. Inactivating mutations at the 17p13 locus including the TP53 tumor suppressor gene and alterations of the 11p15 locus leading to IGF-2 overexpression are frequently observed in ACC. *In vitro* experiments suggest that overexpressed IGF-2 acting via the IGF-1 receptor may play a role in the adrenal cancer cell proliferation.

## CLINICAL PRESENTATION

Approximately half of the patients with ACC have endocrine abnormalities at the time of diagnosis. Children are more likely to present with endocrine abnormalities compared to adults. Rapidly progressing Cushing syndrome is present in 30–40% of patients with ACC. Virilization owing to hypersecretion of adrenal androgens is present in 20–30% of females with ACC (**166**). Feminization in males, hyperaldosteronism, hypoglycemia, and polycythemia are other rare clinical presentations. Patients with no recognizable endocrine syndromes present with abdominal pain, fullness, or an incidentally discovered adrenal mass. A palpable mass is present in approximately half of these patients at the time of diagnosis. Local invasion involving the kidneys and inferior vena cava can be seen in up to 20% of patients. The most common sites of metastases are retroperitoneal lymph nodes, lungs, liver, or bone.

## DIAGNOSIS

### Imaging

The noncontrast CT scan is the preferred initial diagnostic study for suspected ACC. Approximately three-quarters of ACC are more than 6 cm at presentation (**167**). Large tumors commonly demonstrate necrosis or hemorrhage and may contain calcifications. Small lesions may be homogeneous and usually have a noncontrast CT Hounsfield unit (HU) >30. MRI (**168**) is best used for defining local extension of the tumor into the inferior vena cava. PET using FDG shows abnormal tracer uptake in ACC and is helpful in the diagnosis, but is expensive and not widely available.

### Hormonal work-up

The extent of the biochemical evaluation of patients suspected to have ACC depends on the clinical presentation. A pheochromocytoma should be ruled out before surgery in all patients. It is important to screen for hypercortisolism before surgery in order to recognize and treat postoperative adrenal insufficiency, which develops in patients with autonomous cortisol production. High levels of inactive steroid precursors, such as pregnenolone, 17-hydroxy-pregnenolone, 11-deoxycortisol or their metabolites can be found in some patients. An ACC secreting aldosterone precursors like deoxycorticosterone or corticosterone can cause features of hyperaldosteronism. High concentrations of adrenal androgens and androgen precursors like DHEAS and androstenedione in blood are usually seen in patients with virilization.

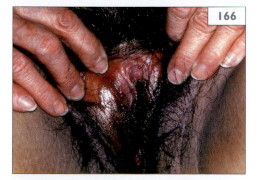

166 Clitoromegaly in a woman with adrenocortical carcinoma secondary to excess androgen secretion. (Courtesy of Dr. Charles Faiman, Department of Endocrinology, Diabetes, and Metabolism, Cleveland Clinic.)

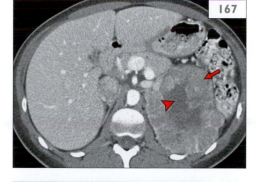

167 CT scan of abdomen with intravenous contrast in a patient with adrenocortical carcinoma showing a 12.6 cm heterogeneous lobulated mass occupying the left renal fossa (arrow). Area of necrosis is seen in the center (arrowhead).

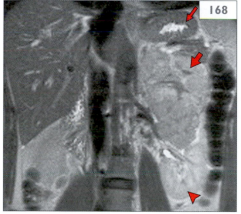

168 Coronal view of T1-weighted gadolinium-enhanced abdominal MRI image of the same patient in 167 showing a large lobulated mass in the left upper quadrant of the abdomen (large arrow) displacing the left kidney inferiorly (arrowhead) and the stomach superiorly (arrow). There is heterogeneous enhancement after giving contrast.

## PATHOLOGY AND STAGING

A diagnosis of ACC is based on both macroscopic (**169**) and microscopic (**170**) features. Large tumor, hemorrhage, local invasion, nuclear atypia, atypical and frequent mitoses, vascular and capsular invasion, and necrosis are features of malignancy. In addition, broad fibrous bands is a characteristic feature distinguishing ACC from benign tumors. Stage I and II describe localized tumors ≤5 cm and >5 cm, respectively. Locally invasive tumors or tumors with regional lymph node metastases are classified as stage III, whereas stage IV consists of tumors invading the adjacent organs or presenting with distant metastases.

## MANAGEMENT/TREATMENT

### Surgery

In stages I–III, complete tumor removal by an experienced surgeon offers the best chance for cure. Surgery often needs to be extensive with 'en bloc' resection of involved organs. The presence of a tumor thrombus in the inferior vena cava or the renal vein is compatible with complete tumor resection but occasionally necessitates cardiac bypass technique. Open adrenalectomy is advised, since the laparoscopic technique is associated with a high risk for local recurrence. Tumor debulking does not improve survival, but may be helpful in controlling the symptoms due to hormonal excess. Surgery for

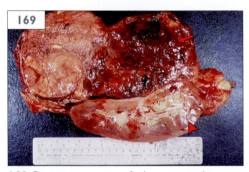

**169** Gross appearance of adrenocortical carcinoma: 15 cm gray-tan and hemorrhagic, variegated tumor totally replacing the adrenal gland (arrow). The normal kidney is seen inferior to the mass (arrowhead). (Courtesy of Dr. Howard Levin, Department of Anatomic Pathology, Cleveland Clinic.)

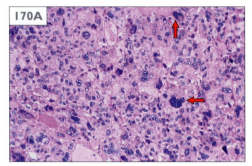

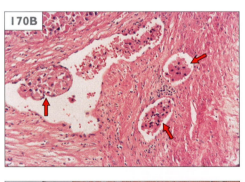

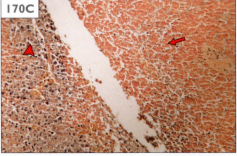

**170** Microscopic appearance of an adrenal cortical carcinoma. **A**: Marked hypercellularity with loss of sinusoidal architecture and marked nuclear pleomorphism (arrows); **B**: vascular invasion: arrows show the presence of carcinomatous cells within three blood vessels; **C**: extensive necrosis (arrow) and focal residual viable adrenal cortical carcinoma cells (arrowhead). (Courtesy of Dr. Howard Levin, Department of Anatomic Pathology, Cleveland Clinic.)

local recurrences or metastatic disease may be associated with improved survival.

## Radiation therapy
Up to 40% of patients with ACC show some response to radiation therapy (RT). RT is useful to control localized disease not amenable to surgery. Adjuvant RT to the tumor bed after complete resection is associated with decreased local recurrence in small studies. RT is useful for symptom control in patients with distant metastases to the bone and brain.

## Medical therapy
Mitotane is the only adrenal-specific agent available for treatment of ACC. It exerts a specific cytolytic effect on adrenocortical cells and inhibits adrenal steroidogenic enzymes. Mitotane leads to an objective tumor regression in about 25% of patients with ACC and controls symptoms of hormone excess in the majority of patients. The dosage of mitotane is adjusted based on tolerability and serum levels. There is a high incidence of gastrointestinal and central nervous system side-effects. In addition, all patients should be placed on glucocorticoids for treatment of adrenal insufficiency induced by mitotane. The use of mitotane as an adjuvant therapy starting soon after surgery may be associated with better long-term outcome.

Combination chemotherapy has minimal success in treatment of ACC. A variety of regimens including vincristine, cisplatin, temiposide and cyclophosphamide (OPEC), and mitotane plus streptozotosin have been tried. Medications like ketoconazole, etomidate, aminoglutethimide, and metyrapone may be used in controlling symptoms of cortisol excess.

## FOLLOW-UP AND PROGNOSIS
Hormonal markers and imaging studies should be done every 3 months after surgery for early detection of tumor recurrence. CT scan of abdomen and chest is the preferred imaging modality.[18]F-FDG PET may be helpful for detecting local recurrence. Prognosis of ACC is poor (mean survival of 18 months) and it depends largely on tumor stage. Aggressive initial surgery followed by initiation of mitotane soon after surgery may increase the median survival in many patients up to 4–5 years. In general, children have a better prognosis than others.

# Adrenal incidentaloma

## DEFINITION
Adrenal incidentaloma (AIn) is an adrenal mass 1 cm or more in diameter that is accidentally discovered by radiologic examination in the absence of symptoms or clinical findings suggestive of adrenal disease. Patients undergoing imaging procedures as a part of staging and work-up for cancer are excluded from this definition.

## PREVALENCE/ETIOLOGY
The prevalence of AIn varies with age and ranges from 1.4 to 8.7%. Incidental adrenal masses are found in 0.5–5% of patients undergoing CT scan of the abdomen. *Table 19* lists the most common causes of AIn and their prevalence.

**Table 19 Causes and prevalence of adrenal incidentalomas**

| Etiology | Prevalence (%) |
|---|---|
| Adrenal cortical tumors | |
| adenoma | 36–94 |
| nodular hyperplasia | 7–17 |
| carcinoma | 0.1–2 |
| Adrenal medullary tumors | |
| pheochromocytoma | 1.5–23 |
| Other adrenal tumors | |
| myelolipoma | 7–15 |
| lipoma | 0–11 |
| Cysts and pseudocysts | 4–22 |
| Hematoma and hemorrhage | 0–4 |
| Infections and granulomas | Rare |
| Metastases | 0–21 |

(From Gopan T, *et al.* 2006. Evaluating and managing adrenal incidentalomas. Cleveland Clinic Journal of Medicine 73;561–8, with permission.)

## DIAGNOSIS

Two questions need to be answered in any case of AIn:
- Is it malignant?
- Is it functional?

### Benign or malignant

Imaging characteristics and tumor size are the two major predictors to differentiate between benign and malignant adrenal masses.

### Imaging studies

The noncontrast CT scan of the adrenals is the best initial imaging study to evaluate an AIn. A maximum noncontrast CT attenuation co-efficient expressed in Hounsfield units ≤10 of an adrenal mass indicates high fat content and has 100% specificity to rule out adrenocortical carcinoma and metastasis (**171–173**). A noncontrast CT HU >10 may be seen in malignant as well as lipid-poor benign adrenal tumors. In such circumstances, measurement of enhancement washout percentage at 15 minutes may help to differentiate between the two. Values less than 60% are suggestive of nonadenomas. Noncontrast CT HU cannot discriminate between the various secretory adrenal tumors, but a value ≤10 makes the diagnosis of pheochromocytoma very unlikely.

MRI imaging characteristics may also be used to differentiate between the benign and malignant adrenal masses. On T1-weighted images, a drop in signal intensity during opposed phase (out-of-phase) compared to in-phase images is consistent with high fat content and is highly specific for benign adrenal masses (**174A, B**).

Adrenal scintigraphy using [131]I-6 beta-iodomethyl-norcholesterol ([131]I-NP-59) has been used to differentiate benign from malignant adrenal masses larger than 2 cm. Increased tracer uptake at the side of the detected mass, has been proposed as a typical pattern of benign cortical adenoma or nodular hyperplasia. In contrast, absent or decreased uptake by the adrenal mass may indicate adrenocortical carcinoma, metastasis, or other nonfunctioning, space-occupying or destructive adrenal lesions. However, this test is not widely available and takes 5–7 days to complete, limiting its useful-ness. PET using FDG shows abnormal tracer uptake in malignant adrenal masses. Although initial reports were promising, FDG PET is more expensive and much less widely available than CT and MRI, and there are few published data on its accuracy to predict its future role in the evaluation of incidental adrenal masses.

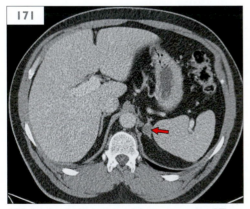

171 A left adrenal mass with noncontrast CT scan HU of –5, which is consistent with a benign adenoma (arrow). (From Gopan T, et al. 2006. Evaluating and managing adrenal incidentalomas. *Cleveland Clinic Journal of Medicine* **73**;561–8, with permission.)

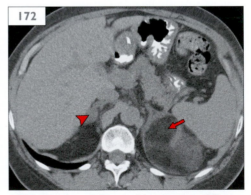

172 Adrenal myelolipoma. Noncontrast CT scan image of a left adrenal myelolipoma. The lesion appears heterogeneous, with areas of very low Hounsfield Units (<–30) due to the high fat content (arrow). A right adrenal adenoma is also seen (arrowhead).

## Tumor size

The probability of an adrenal mass being malignant increases with its size. Once imaging characteristics are taken into consideration, a 6-cm tumor size is a reasonable cut-off for surgical resection. With a few exceptions, the lack of change in the size of an adrenal mass (<1 cm) over 6–12 months is suggestive of a benign nature.

## Fine-needle aspiration

Image-guided FNA may be helpful in the diagnostic evaluation of patients with known extra-adrenal primary malignancy and a newly discovered adrenal mass with a noncontrast CT attenuation value >10 HU. A pheochromocytoma should always be excluded before FNA of an adrenal mass is attempted to avoid the potential risk for a hypertensive crisis. FNA may not differentiate adrenocortical carcinoma from an adrenal adenoma.

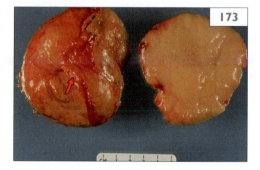

**173** Gross specimen of an adrenal myelolipoma: 7.5 cm bivalved yellow mass is shown. Normal adrenal cortex is splayed over the surface (arrow). (Courtesy of Dr. Howard Levin, Department of Anatomic Pathology, Cleveland Clinic.)

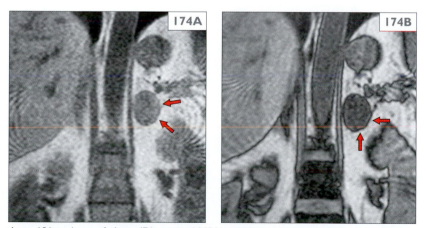

**174** In-phase (**A**) and out of phase (**B**) coronal MRI image in a patient with left adrenal mass (arrows). There is a decrease in signal intensity of the mass in the out of phase image due to high fat content, which is consistent with adenoma/hyperplasia. (From Gopan T, *et al.* 2006. Evaluating and managing adrenal incidentalomas. *Cleveland Clinic Journal of Medicine* **73**;561–8, with permission.)

## Hormonal evaluation

The overall prevalence of hormonal abnormalities in AIn ranges from 6 to 24%. All patients with AIn should undergo evaluation for the following conditions at a minimum:

- Pheochromocytoma.
- Cushing syndrome.
- Primary aldosteronism (only if hypertensive).

## Pheochromocytoma

Screening for pheochromocytoma is mandatory in all cases of AIn since this condition may be associated with significant morbidity and mortality with an unpredictable course. It could be completely asymptomatic in up to 15% of patients. The measurement of plasma metanephrines or 24-hour urine metanephrines are appropriate initial screening tests (see Pheochromocytoma, page 130).

## Cushing syndrome

Most patients with cortisol-secreting AIn do not have the typical signs and symptoms associated with CS. Instead, they may have a relatively recent and poorly described disorder known as subclinical Cushing syndrome (SCS). Such patients develop adrenal insufficiency following the resection of adrenal tumor due to chronic suppression of the contralateral adrenal gland. Overnight 1 mg dexamethasone suppression test (DST) is the initial screening test of choice. A serum cortisol value >138 nmol/L (5 µg/dL) during 1 mg DST and a low or suppressed ACTH level (preferably AM) strongly supports the diagnosis of SCS. A cortisol value <50 nmol/L (1.8 µg/dL) during 1 mg DST makes the diagnosis unlikely. Patients with indeterminate cortisol levels may further be evaluated by measuring 24-hour urine free cortisol, midnight salivary cortisol, and the CRH stimulation test.

## Primary aldosteronism

Only hypertensive patients with AIn should be evaluated for primary aldosteronism. The best initial screening test is the ambulatory PAC to PRA ratio. A PAC (pmol/L)/PRA (ng/mL/h) ratio of 555 (20, if aldosterone is expressed as ng/dL) or greater with a concomitant PAC above 275 pmol/L (10 ng/dL) needs to be pursued further by measurement of 24-hour urine aldosterone during salt loading (see Primary aldosteronism, page X).

## Other hormonal evaluation

Women with adrenal mass and physical findings suggestive of hyperandrogenism should have their total testosterone and DHEAS levels measured. Routine screening for androgen excess in patients with AIn in the absence of suggestive clinical features is not warranted.

## EVALUATION/MANAGEMENT

An approach to incidentally discovered adrenal masses is shown in **175**. Adrenal masses with a maximum noncontrast CT HU ≤10 are benign and do not require any routine follow-up imaging study. Such patients, especially those with an adrenal mass >3 cm, should undergo annual evaluation for hormonal hypersecretion. The optimal duration of follow-up is not known. The patients with a noncontrast CT HU >10 and tumor size >6 cm should be referred for surgery. Those with a noncontrast CT HU >10 and tumor size <6 cm should have the delayed enhancement washout percentage at 15 minutes calculated and have follow-up imaging study in 6–12 months. There is no good evidence supporting continued radiologic surveillance if the follow up study at 6–12 months shows no significant change (<1 cm) in the adrenal tumor size.

## Surgery

Laparoscopic adrenalectomy is the treatment of choice for most adrenal masses, which are functional or malignant. Medical therapy may be acceptable in the case of primary hyperaldosteronism secondary to adrenocortical adenoma/hyperplasia. Surgery in those with widespread malignancy is usually not indicated. Compared to open adrenalectomy, the laparoscopic approach is associated with decreased postoperative pain, reduced time to return of bowel function, decreased length of hospital stay, and the potential for earlier return to work.

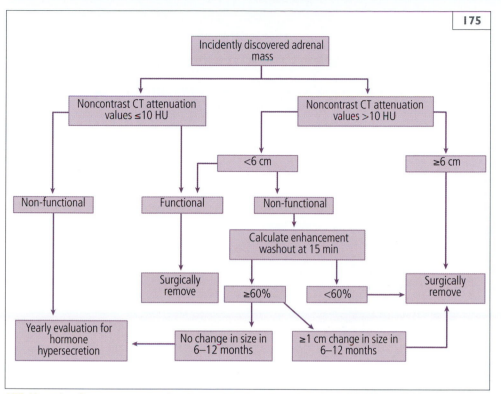

**175** Algorithm for management of patients with adrenal incidentaloma. HU: Hounsfield unit. (From Gopan T, *et al.* 2006. Evaluating and managing adrenal incidentalomas. *Cleveland Clinic Journal of Medicine* **73**;561–8, with permission.)

# Female and male reproductive disorders

Rhoda Cobin

Rebecca Fenichel

**Polycystic ovary syndrome**

**Female infertility**

**Hyperprolactinemia**

**Secondary amenorrhea**

**Primary amenorrhea**

**Menopause**

**Male infertility**

**Male hypogonadism**

**Gynecomastia**

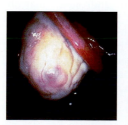 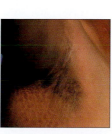 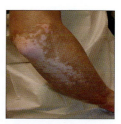

# Polycystic ovary syndrome

## DEFINITION/OVERVIEW

Polycystic ovary syndrome (PCOS) is the most common endocrine disorder of females of reproductive age and the most common cause of menstrual irregularity, occurring in as many as 10% of women in this age group. Various definitions have been proposed to confirm the diagnosis. The Rotterdam conference proposed that two of three criteria must be present including polycystic ovaries on ultrasound, oligo- or anovulation, and hyperandrogenism, while a National Institutes of Health (NIH) consensus concluded that the sonographic findings may not be required to make the diagnosis. Some authorities note that many women actually have regular menses, but have hyperandrogenism and sonographically normal ovaries. Obviously with such variable definitions, the diagnosis is often one of exclusion of other disorders presenting with oligomenorrhea, anovulation, or hyperandrogenism (see below).

The etiology of PCOS is poorly understood. There is genetic clustering of this disorder and a strong association with the insulin resistance syndrome. Various candidate genes have been proposed but none have been definitively found to be causative.

## PATHOPHYSIOLOGY

In the ovary, there is abnormal steroidogenesis resulting in excess production of ovarian androgens including testosterone and androstenedione. There is abnormal hypothalamic regulation suggesting disordered dopaminergic input, with tonically elevated acyclic LH release and relatively low FSH. Whether this is causal or a result of the effects of ovarian hyperandrogenism is still unknown.

The morphologic characteristics of the ovaries include multiple macro- and microscopic peripheral cysts (**176**) along with a variable degree of stromal or thecal hyperplasia. The ovaries may or may not be increased in overall size. The finding of insulin resistance in a majority of females with PCOS has led to a more unifying hypothesis suggesting that the resulting hyperinsulinism causes excess androgen production with secondary hypothalamic dysfunction. The efficacy of insulin sensitizers in restoring regular ovulation even in females without overt insulin resistance would support this notion.

## CLINICAL PRESENTATION

While PCOS typically presents with oligomenorrhea present from the time of menarche, along with signs of hyperandrogenism including hirsutism (**177**) acne (**178**) acanthosis (**179**) and often alopecia, some women present later, often with anovulatory infertility. Girls with precocious pubarche often develop PCOS later in life. Individuals may have any or all of the clinical findings at various times in their lives. Generally, very severe hyperandrogenism (virilization including baldness, clitoromegaly, and muscle hypertrophy) (**180**) would suggest disorders other than PCOS.

## DIFFERENTIAL DIAGNOSIS

This includes late-onset adrenal hyperplasia (21-hydroxylase deficiency or less commonly 11-hydroxylase deficiency), ovarian and adrenal androgen-producing tumors, hyperthecosis ovarii, and CS. There is considerable overlap with a condition labeled idiopathic hirsutism. Genetic and ethnic variations in normal body hair distribution complicate the picture.

## DIAGNOSIS

The diagnosis of PCOS is one of exclusion of the conditions listed above. A LH/FSH ratio over 2.5–3 is suggestive, as are testosterone/androstenedione levels in the 'high-normal' to moderately elevated range. (Since steroid assays in this range are extremely difficult and somewhat unreliable, clinical presentation is very important). Testosterone levels above 150–200 ng/dL would suggest tumor. DHEAS, an adrenal androgen, may be modestly elevated. In addition to the measurement of gonadotropins and androgens, cortisol, sex steroid-binding globulin, 17-alpha-hydroxyprogesterone, PRL, and thyroid tests should be performed to exclude other common causes of menstrual irregularity and hyperandrogenism.

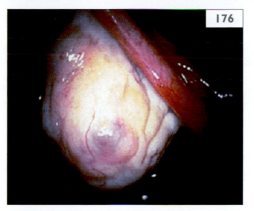

176 Gross picture of polycystic ovaries.
(Courtesy of Dr. Michael Zinaman.)

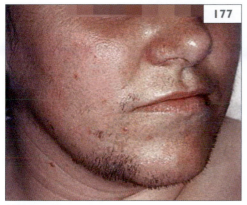

177 Facial hirsutism.

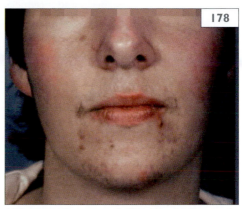

178 Acne. (Courtesy of of Dr. Donald Gordon.)

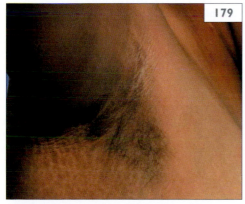

179 Acanthosis nigricans. (Courtesy of Dr.
Donald Gordon.)

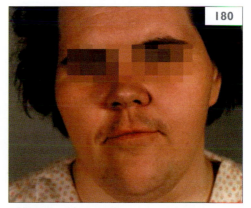

180 Virilized female. (Courtesy of of Dr. Donald
Gordon.)

Because of the strong association of PCOS and insulin resistance and the excess risk of type 2 diabetes mellitus, hypertension, stroke, and myocardial infarction, it is important to assess blood pressure, lipids, glucose (2 hr post glucose is a more sensitive marker of insulin resistance than FBS). Some authorities suggest that inflammatory markers and 'nontraditional risk factors' also be measured.

## MANAGEMENT/TREATMENT

Therapy for PCOS depends upon the time in a woman's life, as well as her current treatment goals. 80% of women will have restoration of regular ovulatory menses with metformin, making this the drug of choice for those who wish to achieve pregnancy. Since this agent reduces insulin resistance and reduces progression to overt diabetes, its metabolic effects are beneficial. Thiazolidendiones are also effective but are Category C drugs for pregnancy. Excess androgen may not be as reliably suppressed using insulin sensitizers and may require ovarian suppression with OCPs, noting that these agents may exacerbate insulin resistance. Antiandrogens including spirono-lactone and flutamide may also be required to reduce hirsutism, and the topical agent eflorni-thine, an ornithine decarboxylase inhibitor) may be a useful adjunct.

# Female infertility

## DEFINITION/OVERVIEW

Infertility is defined as an inability to conceive after 12 months of frequent intercourse, given that no contraception is used. Infertility can be related to a male factor, female factor, or in many cases both partners are affected.

## ETIOLOGY

The etiology of female infertility can be divided into disorders of the follicle, fallopian tubes, and uterus, as well as hormonal problems including disorders of the hypothalamic–pituitary–ovarian (HPO) axis and endomet-rium. Chronic diseases, such as liver or kidney failure, can also cause infertility.

## PATHOPHYSIOLOGY
### Disorders of ovulation

Ovulation requires an intact HPO axis. Pituitary disorders such as hyperprolactinemia can cause anovulation. If the patient is ovulating, both the quantity and quality of follicles are important determinants of fertility. As females age, the quantity and quality of available follicles decline. This generally coincides with a minimal elevation in FSH when measured on day 3 of the menstrual cycle. Higher FSH levels can signify premature ovarian failure (POF) secondary to toxic exposures (such as to chemotherapy), auto-immune endocrinopathies, or genetic abnor-malities (see section on menopause) such as in the polyglandular syndromes.

### Disorders of the uterus and fallopian tubes

Once it is confirmed that the patient is ovulating, there are common problems that can affect the transfer and implantation of the fertilized egg. A history of previous infection, cyclic pelvic pain, or surgery may reveal the diagnosis. Endometriosis, the presence of endometrial lining cells outside the uterus, and pelvic inflammatory disease, usually caused by infections with *Chlamydia* or *Gonorrhea*, can cause tubal blockages. Adhesions outside the uterus are a common problem, and can occur after a severe abdominal infection or prior surgery, and affect the transfer of the fertilized egg to the uterine lining. Inside the uterus, structural problems such as submucosal fibroids, synechiae due to prior surgery, or endometrial polyps can prevent implantation. Though uncommon, uterine anomalies can be associated with infertility. These include the septate or bicornuate uterus. Assisted reproduction may be required, but most patients can ultimately conceive.

### Disorders of the endometrium

During the second half of the menstrual cycle, progesterone exposure matures the endometrium and readies it for implantation. Though it is difficult to measure and its significance is unclear, some females exhibit a delayed maturation of the endometrial lining. This is commonly referred to as a luteal phase defect, and may represent inadequate progesterone secretion by the corpus luteum.

### DIAGNOSIS

For the work-up of female infertility, the first stage is to document whether the patient is ovulating. Even in the presence of reported monthly bleeding, ovulation may not be occurring. Ovulation can be documented by a daily temperature chart, with home measurement of the LH surge with urine kits, or by checking progesterone levels during the second half of the menstrual cycle. If the patient is not ovulating, hormonal disturbances such as hyperprolactinemia, thyroid dysfunction, PCOS, and hypogonadotropic hypogonadism should be ruled out, and FSH should be tested on day 3 of the menstrual cycle to evaluate the quality and quantity of available follicles. A karyotype can also be performed to rule out genetic syndromes that may present with infertility such as Turner's syndrome (specifically XO/XX mosaicism).

Fibroids and polyps can be seen on transvaginal ultrasound, while tubal blockage can be diagnosed with a hysterosalpingogram (**181**). Endometriosis can be diagnosed on laparoscopy, or sometimes on transvaginal ultrasound in the form of endometriomas ('chocolate cysts') on the ovary. Luteal phase defects can be suggested by lower progesterone levels during the luteal phase and, in some cases, an endometrial biopsy is required.

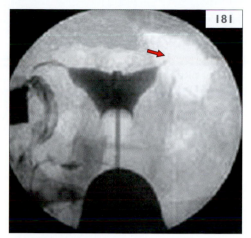

**181** Hysterosalpingogram showing a blocked fallopian tube (arrow). (From www.centerforhumanreprod.com/treat_gyne.html, with permission.)

### MANAGEMENT/TREATMENT

Treatment of anovulation should be directed to the underlying problem. In some patients, ovulation can be induced by correcting the underlying hormonal disturbance (such as with insulin sensitizers in patients with PCOS). If therapy is unsuccessful, ovulation induction with clomiphene citrate or exogenous gonadotropins can be tried. If infertility persists, the next step is usually *in vitro* fertilization. Patients with POF can become pregnant through egg donation programs.

Structural problems with the uterus or fallopian tubes can be treated surgically or overcome with *in vitro* fertilization. Endometriosis can be treated at the time of laparoscopy, although it is uncertain whether this improves fertility.

# Hyperprolactinemia

## DEFINITION/OVERVIEW

Prolactin is a peptide hormone secreted by the anterior pituitary gland. Its main physiologic role is to promote milk secretion. Therefore, PRL is normally elevated during pregnancy and lactation. Any elevation outside the normal range is considered significant; however, the extent of elevation may provide a clue to the etiology of hyperprolactinemia. A persistently elevated PRL level should prompt investigation.

## ETIOLOGY

PRL secretion is regulated by tonic inhibition by dopamine from the hypothalamus. Therefore, high PRL levels may be due to autonomously functioning pituitary tissue, or by anything that lowers dopamine inhibition of PRL secretion.

## PATHOGENESIS
### Pituitary tumors

Pituitary tumors are common, and prolactinomas are the most common type of secretory pituitary tumor. However, any sellar lesion or injury that is significant enough to affect the hypothalamus or the hypothalamic–pituitary stalk can cause hyperprolactinemia due to decreased dopamine inhibition of PRL secretion ('stalk effect'). These can include craniopharyngiomas, metastatic disease, infiltrative diseases, or any other pituitary adenoma.

### Iatrogenic hyperprolactinemia

There are many medications that inhibit the dopamine system, and therefore decrease inhibition of PRL secretion. These include several antipsychotics, antidepressants, antihypertensives, protease inhibitors, and some antiemetics.

### Idiopathic hyperprolactinemia

In some patients, a cause cannot be found. Many of these patients may harbor small microprolactinomas that are not visible on imaging studies. Most of these patients do not progress, but should be monitored.

## CLINICAL PRESENTATION

Patients may present with spontaneous or expressive galactorrhea. In women, hyperprolactinemia can present as a hypoestrogenic state including menstrual dysfunction and vaginal dryness. In males, hyperprolactinemia can present with hypogonadism causing decreased libido and energy, and eventually loss of sexual hair, osteoporosis, and loss of muscle mass. It can also cause erectile dysfunction despite normal testosterone levels via an unknown mechanism.

## DIFFERENTIAL DIAGNOSIS

The differential diagnosis of a high PRL level therefore includes disorders of the pituitary gland (functioning and nonfunctioning adenomas), medication-induced hyperprolactinemia, and idiopathic hyperprolactinemia. Minimal elevations in PRL can also be seen in other endocrine disorders including PCOS and hypothyroidism (due to TRH stimulation). PRL levels can also be transiently elevated due to nipple stimulation, stress, and exercise, or due to chest wall injury. Finally, PRL can be elevated in patients with decreased PRL clearance. This can occur in patients with chronic renal failure and, rarely, in patients who secrete high levels of glycosylated PRL which circulates in aggregates and prevents renal clearance ('macroprolactinemia').

If PRL is found to be elevated, the test should be repeated. Unless a patient is on a medication known to cause hyperprolactinemia, an MRI of the pituitary should be performed. PRL levels below 200 ng/mL can be related to any of the above causes. However, levels above 200 ng/mL are most consistent with a pituitary macroadenoma (**182A, B**). Conversely, if a macroadenoma is present but the PRL level is curiously low, serum PRL should be measured with serial dilutions to rule out a 'hook effect' which is caused by very high PRL levels which overwhelm the commonly used assay for this hormone.

## MANAGEMENT/TREATMENT

Dopamine agonists (cabergoline or bromo-criptine) can be used to treat all causes of hyperprolactinemia when indicated. Cabergoline is usually first-line therapy due to its longer duration of action and more favorable side-effect profile. PRL levels should be followed to evaluate the response to therapy. Asymptomatic hyperprolactinemia that is not due to a pituitary macroadenoma does not always require treatment. Galactorrhea requires treatment only if it is bothersome to the patient. However, hyperprolactinemia with consequent hypogonadism should always be treated if possible to prevent bone loss. If a patient has iatrogenic hyperprolactinemia and medications cannot be substituted, sex steroid hormone replacement is an alternative.

Dopamine agonists can also be used to treat prolactinomas effectively. Symptomatic microprolactinomas (<1 cm), as well as all macroprolactinomas (>1 cm), should be treated with dopamine receptor agonists. Specifically, macroprolactinomas of all sizes should be treated to prevent visual loss due to enlargement of the adenoma towards the optic chiasm. If medications are ineffective, transsphenoidal surgery should be considered.

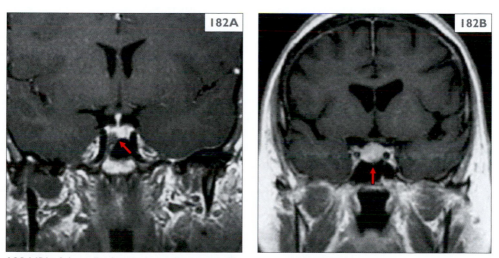

182 MRI of the sella showing a prolactinoma. (From Schlechte JA [2003]. Prolactinoma. *N Engl J Med* **349**:2035–2041. Copyright 2003 Massachusetts Medical Society. All rights reserved..)

# Secondary amenorrhea

## DEFINITION/OVERVIEW

Amenorrhea is defined as the absence of menses. Depending on the timing of presentation, amenorrhea can be divided into primary and secondary amenorrhea. Primary amenorrhea, which is discussed in the next section, refers to an absence of menarche by age 15. Secondary amenorrhea refers to a cessation of menses after menarche, and is considered clinically significant if the amenorrhea lasts for more than 3 months or the patient misses more than three cycles during any given year. The most common causes of secondary amenorrhea are physiologic and include pregnancy and lactation.

## ETIOLOGY

Amenorrhea can be due to disorders of the hypothalamus, pituitary, ovary, and uterus. Aside from pregnancy, the most common causes of secondary amenorrhea are PCOS, hypothalamic amenorrhea, hyperprolactinemia, and POF. PCOS and hyperprolactinemia are discussed elsewhere in this chapter.

## PATHOGENESIS

Hypothalamic amenorrhea is a characterized by decreased or disordered GnRH secretion or pulsatility. This leads to altered LH pulsatility, low gonadotropin levels, and a hypoestrogenic state. In many cases, this condition is associated with either a physical or psychologic stressor, but in some cases no cause is found. Most commonly, there is a history of intense exercise or caloric restriction, which results in a negative energy balance and may be associated with low body weight (often 10% below ideal), low fat mass, and low leptin levels. Emotional stress and chronic illness can cause a similar picture. In these cases, LH, FSH, and estradiol levels are low, and MRI imaging reveals no pituitary or hypothalamic disease.

There are several ways in which pituitary disease can cause amenorrhea. Aside from prolactinomas, ACTH-secreting adenomas causing CS can also cause amenorrhea. This can be confirmed with measurement of 24-hour urine free cortisol. Other sellar lesions (cysts, craniopharyngiomas) large enough to compromise normal pituitary function can cause secondary hypogonadism. Infiltrative diseases may include sarcoidosis and lymphocytic hypophysitis. Sheehan's syndrome (pituitary infarction most commonly seen after pregnancy) or radiation may lead to empty sella syndrome and consequent hypogonadism.

Ovulatory disorders can be caused by PCOS or other hyperandrogenic disorders, or ovarian failure. POF is a depletion of ovarian follicles before age 40. These females have low estradiol levels but elevated gonadotropins due to the loss of negative feedback by estrogen and inhibins. Elevated FSH levels distinguish this syndrome from hypothalamic amenorrhea in females of reproductive age. POF can be due to toxic exposures (such as chemotherapy), genetic abnormalities (such as Turner's 45XO/45XX mosaicism and Fragile X), smoking, or polyglandular autoimmune disease. Asherman's syndrome due to scarring of the uterus from previous surgery can also cause secondary amenorrhea.

## CLINICAL PRESENTATION/ DIFFERENTIAL DIAGNOSIS

Women may present with oligomenorrhea or, if prolonged, with hypoestrogenism. Baseline laboratory testing should include serum hCG to rule out pregnancy, estradiol, FSH, PRL, and TSH levels. Medications should be reviewed. A history of over-exercising or eating disorders accompanied by a low body mass index suggests hypothalamic amenorrhea. If there is evidence of hirsutism, male pattern hair loss, acne, or signs of metabolic syndrome on exam, PCOS should be considered. Striae, muscle weakness, central obesity, easy bruising, or hypertension suggest Cushing's disease. Headaches, visual changes or the presence of multiple pituitary deficiencies suggests a space-occupying sellar lesion or pituitary infiltrative disease. A history of hypothyroidism, vitiligo (**183A, B**), adrenal insufficiency, or diabetes suggests autoimmune POF. Antithyroid peroxidase, antithyroglobulin, or antiadrenal antibodies can clarify the diagnosis. Turner's mosaicism and other genetic abnormalities can be revealed by karyotype analysis.

## MANAGEMENT/TREATMENT

Patients with hypothalamic amenorrhea can recover with treatment of the underlying stressor, for example with weight gain. It is important that any hormonal and nutritional deficiencies be corrected, because even at a young age, these patients are at risk for low bone density and fractures. If fertility is an issue, gonadotropins can be used.

The diagnosis of POF is a difficult one for both the physician and the patient. Patients will require sex steroid replacement for both bone health and quality of life issues. The treatment of PCOS and hyperprolactinemia is discussed elsewhere in this chapter.

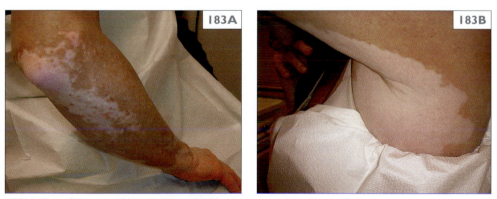

**183** Vitiligo of the arm (**A**) and abdomen (**B**). (Courtesy of Dr. Rhoda Cobin.)

# Primary amenorrhea

### DEFINITION/OVERVIEW

Primary amenorrhea refers to an absence of menarche by age 15. The absence of menarche should be considered in the context of a patient's personal and family history of pubertal development. In general, disorders that exclusively cause primary amenorrhea are relatively uncommon. However, most disorders that cause secondary amenorrhea can also cause primary amenorrhea.

### ETIOLOGY/PATHOGENESIS

Primary amenorrhea can be due to disorders of the hypothalamus, pituitary, ovary, uterus, or outflow tract. Pituitary disease, such as hyper-prolactinemia and hypothalamic amenorrhea, account for about 20% of cases. In addition to these more common hormonal disorders, a number of genetic and anatomic abnormalities must be considered in a patient presenting with primary amenorrhea. In general, patients are affected by either gonadal failure or by a congenital lesion of the reproductive tract.

Primary gonadal failure (or gonadal dysgenesis, 'streak gonad') in which fibrosis occurs and follicles are depleted, may occur at any point in time, even *in utero*. These account for about 50% of cases of primary amenorrhea. The most common type of gonadal dysgenesis is Turner's syndrome (gonadal dysgenesis due to 45XO karyotype or mosaicism). These patients often present long before puberty with well-known clinical stigmata including short stature, webbed neck, low hairline, and shield chest (**184, 185A–C**). Very early gonadal failure in patients with 45XY genotype can also occur ('vanishing testes syndrome') resulting in female external genitalia but lacking mullerian structures due to the presence of mullerian-inhibiting hormone. Secondary gonadal failure due to congential GnRH deficiency may also occur, often in conjunction with anosmia (Kallman's syndrome).

Though rare, other disorders associated with a male genotype (46XY) but female phenotype include absent testis-determining factor, androgen insensitivity, adrenal enzyme deficiencies (such as 17-alpha hydroxylase deficiency), LH receptor defects, and aromatase deficiency. Androgen insensitivity can be suspected on physical examination and easily distinguished by very high testosterone levels (**186**). Congenital lesions of the uterus and vagina cause approximately 20% of cases. These include imperforate hymen (**187**), vaginal septae, and mullerian agenesis, which can affect the vagina and sometimes the uterus.

### CLINICAL PRESENTATION/ DIFFERENTIAL DIAGNOSIS

A careful history should be taken with regard to puberty and family history. The patient should be examined for evidence of previous estrogen exposure (breast development), axillary and pubic hair, as well as stigmata of Turner's syndrome. Pelvic examination can reveal clitoromegaly, an imperforate hymen, transverse vaginal septum, or partial or complete agenesis of the vagina and/or uterus. A history of cyclic pelvic pain or perirectal mass (representing the sequestration of blood in the pelvis) suggests an anatomic abnormality preventing menstrual blood flow.

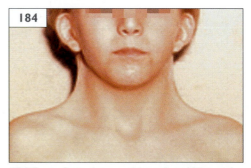

**184** Turner's syndrome with neck webbing and shield chest. (Courtesy of Dr. Donald Gordon.)

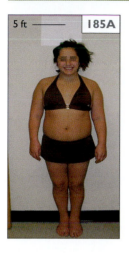

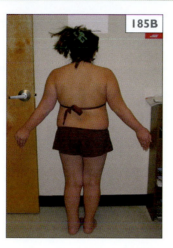

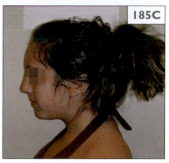

185 Turner's syndrome. **A**: Short stature; **B**: increased carrying angle in the upper extremities; **C**: Low set ears. (Courtesy of Dr. Rhoda Cobin.)

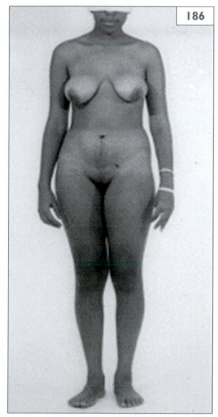

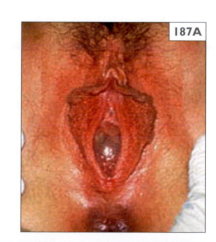

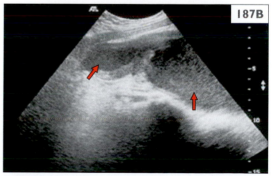

186 Androgen insensitivity syndrome. (Courtesy of Dr. Donald Gordon.)

187 Imperforate hymen. (From Stone SM, Alexander JL [2004]. Images in clinical medicine. Imperforate hymen with hematocolpometra. *N Engl J Med* **351**(7):e6. Copyright 2004 Massachusetts Medical Society. All rights reserved.)

## DIFFERENTIAL DIAGNOSIS

Patients with primary amenorrhea should be examined for evidence of secondary sex characteristics and the presence of mullerian structures (vagina, cervix, and uterus). If a pelvic examination cannot be performed, transabdominal ultrasound can be used to visualize mullerian structures. If the uterus is absent, a karyotype along with testosterone levels will help distinguish between mullerian agenesis (45XX) and androgen insensitivity (45XY). If the uterus is present, the cause for gonadal failure should be sought. Low gonadotropin levels suggests a hypothalamic or pituitary cause (hypothalamic amenorrhea, Kallman's syndrome, pituitary failure, hyperprolactinemia, or infiltrative disease). In these cases, pituitary MRI imaging should be performed. High gonadotropin levels suggest primary ovarian failure. A karyotype may reveal the diagnosis.

## MANAGEMENT/TREATMENT

Many of these disorders have both immediate psychosocial implications and long-term health consequences, requiring an interdisciplinary approach. The treatment of primary amenorrhea includes surgical treatment of any anatomic abnormalities, and long-term sex steroid replacement in cases of gonadal failure. Estrogen and cyclic progesterone replacement can be given to induce normal pubertal changes, and treatment with GH may be necessary to achieve normal height. In patients with gonadal dysgenesis, estrogen replacement should be continued until age 50 to maintain bone health, with progesterone to prevent endometrial hyperplasia. Patients with Turner's syndrome are at risk for hypertension, hypothyroidism, hearing loss, and coarctation of the aorta and should be closely followed. Finally, patients with evidence of Y chromatin must have all gonadal tissue removed due to an increased risk of malignancy.

# Menopause

## DEFINITION/OVERVIEW

Menopause is defined as the physiologic cessation of menses for 1 year. In fact, ovarian estrogen production declines gradually and many women experience symptoms of estrogen deficiency even before menses cease. Normal menopause may occur at any time between the ages of 40 and 50 years of age. POF is defined as occurring before the age of 40 and may either be physiologic or pathologic. Many women will spend at least one-third of their lives in menopause. The consequences of estrogen deficiency may be difficult to separate from the consequences of aging, and both may produce pathology that requires both prevention and therapy.

## ETIOLOGY

Menopause is a normal physiologic event. POF may be a hereditary physiologic event or may occur as a consequence of either genetic disorders most on the X chromosome, including fragile X syndrome or autoimmune oophoritis.

## PATHOPHYSIOLOGY

Menopause is characterized by failure of ovulation and ovarian steroid production. There is loss of ovarian inhibin, which regulates pituitary FSH secretion. Oocyte depletion is seen in the ovary and stromal tissue undergoes normal atrophy.

## CLINICAL PRESENTATION

Patients may present with hot flashes, nocturnal warmth or flushing, disturbed sleep patterns, and vaginal dryness and dyspareunia in addition to menstrual irregularity and eventual amenorrhea. Asymptomatic consequences of estrogen deficiency include osteoporosis and alterations in lipid metabolism. The increased risk of myocardial infarction and stroke as a woman ages are debatably a consequence of estrogen deficiency as well.

## DIFFERENTIAL DIAGNOSIS

The differential diagnosis of menopause is that of all causes of secondary amenorrhea.

## DIAGNOSIS

Elevated FSH levels due to lack of ovarian inhibin are the hallmark of ovarian failure. If it occurs during a normal physiologic time period, no further evaluation is necessary. If ovarian failure is premature, consideration of chromosomal analysis, especially for fragile X syndrome should be considered. Ovarian antibodies in high titers are specific but not very sensitive for autoimmune oophoritis, which may occur in association with other auto-immune disorders or within a family setting.

## MANAGEMENT/TREATMENT

The management of menopause is directed at both amelioration of acute symptoms of estrogen withdrawal (flushing, sleep disturbance, vaginal dryness) and preventive strategies to prevent osteoporosis and other chronic disorders of the aging female, particularly cardiovascular disease.

In the past, estrogen therapy had been considered useful not only in ameliorating the symptoms listed above, but was felt to reduce the risk of myocardial infarction and possibly dementia. In the Womens' Health Initiative study, however, no cardiovascular benefit was found, and therefore, curent guidelines suggest estrogen treatment at the lowest effective dose in the early years of menopause for relief of symptoms for the shortest time possible. Nonestrogenic agents including clonidine, neurontin, SSRIs, and atropinic agents may be useful, although not as effective as estrogen in reducing symptoms when estrogen is contraindicated.

Cardiovascular disease prevention in menopausal women should include appropriate diet, exercise, aggressive management of hyperlipidemia, diabetes, and hypertension, as well as smoking cessation. Osteoporosis therapy when estrogen is not used consists of calcium and vitamin D supplementation and exercise. Pharmacologic agents to be considered include selective estrogen receptor modulators (SERMs), bisphosphonates, and parathyroid hormone.

# Male infertility

## DEFINITION/OVERVIEW
Infertility is defined as a failure of conception by a couple who have been having regular unprotected intercourse for more that 1 year.

## ETIOLOGY
At least 20% of cases of infertility involve both male and female factors. Male infertility results from inadequate sperm production or transport or qualitative abnormalities of the sperm.

## PATHOPHYSIOLOGY
The production of normal sperm requires normal seminiferous tubular function, supported by high levels of intratesticular testosterone, and normal duct system. Cryptorchidism, varicocele, and disorders of sperm motility may cause infertility.

## CLINICAL PRESENTATION
Infertility may occur in otherwise normally virilized men or may occur in conjunction with hypogonadism.

## DIFFERENTIAL DIAGNOSIS
The differential diagnosis includes all disorders causing male hypogonadism, either primary or secondary, as well as disorders which affect only the seminiferous tubule (e.g. 'Sertoli cell only syndrome'.) In cases of azospermia, it is important to exclude obstructive causes where sperm production is actually normal.

## DIAGNOSIS
Semen analysis will demonstrate abnormal sperm count and motility. If this is found, it is important to determine whether hypogonadism is also present and requires therapy. Testicular biopsy may occasionally be required in cases of azospermia.

## MANAGEMENT/TREATMENT
In cases of hypothalamic hypogonadism, pulsatile GnRH therapy has been reported to result in spermatogenesis. Therapy with gonadotropins or their analogs may also be successful. Surgical correction of varicocele has been reported to improve fertility. In the case of testicular failure or functionally abnormal spermatogenesis, such therapy is not useful. Using *in vitro* fertilization techniques, however, use of even a single isolated normal sperm may result in production of viable embryos.

# Male hypogonadism

### DEFINITION/OVERVIEW

Inadequate production or action of androgens in the male is termed hypogonadism. Hypogonadism in the male may be either congenital or acquired, and be due either to primary testicular dysfunction or secondary to impaired gonadotropin stimulation of the testis.

### ETIOLOGY/PATHOPHYSIOLOGY

Normal male development and function depend on the differentiation of the primordial gonad that requires the presence of testis differentiating factors (SRY gene present on the Y chromosome and other transcriptional regulators). The male testis secretes testosterone, a product of the Leydig cells, and produces sperm in the seminiferous tubules. Testosterone is converted either to estrogen or to dihydrotestosterone which binds and activates androgen receptors in target tissues. Regulation of testicular function is by pituitary LH (Leydig cells) and FSH (seminiferous tubules). Hypothalmic GnRH controls pituitary gonadotroph function and in turn, hypothalamic–pituitary secretion is regulated by feedback control including DHT, E2, T, and inhibin, a product of the seminiferous tubules. Male hypogonadism may occur as a result of defects in development or action at any of these sites.

### DIFFERENTIAL DIAGNOSIS

The most common etiology of congenital testicular hypogonadism is Kleinfelter's syndrome, which is due to genetic abnormalities, most often XXY, although other variations including mosaic forms occur. This condition is characterized by androgen deficiency of variable degree, gynecomastia, eunuchoidal proportions, and oligo/azospermia (**188A, B** *overleaf*). Anorchidism, cryptorchism with testicular failure, and testicular regression syndrome may rarely account for failure of testicular function.

Enzymatic deficiencies leading to reduced testosterone production may cause congenital inadequate virilization. Reduction in the level of 5-alpha-reductase enzyme diminishes the conversion of testosterone to dihydrotestosterone which results in inadequate virilization in the prepubertal period with improvement at the time of puberty. Disorders of testosterone action (partial androgen insensitivity syndrome) result from genetic abnormalities in the testosterone receptor and produce variable degrees of incomplete virilization present at birth.

Acquired testicular failure may result from infection (e.g. mumps, HIV), trauma, testicular torsion, chemical (including chemotherapy) or thermal injury, and radiation. Muscular dystrophy may also cause testicular failure. 'Andropause' is the term used when otherwise normal men develop androgen deficiency disproportionate to normal age-related testosterone reduction. Testosterone replacement may be indicated.

The most common form of congenital secondary hypogonadism is Kallman's syndrome, where the absence of the KAL gene (Xp22.3) leads to failure of migration of GnRH neurons from the olfactory area to the hypothalamus resulting in hypothalamic hypogonadism and variable degrees of anosmia. Other congenital disorders causing secondary hypogonadism include Prader–Willi syndrome, Laurence–Moon–Biedel syndrome, generalized congenital hypothalamic deficiency which presents with microphallus and neonatal hypoglycemia, and midline craniofacial developmental defects.

Acquired pituitary disease is usually the result of pituitary tumors, craniopharyngomas, radiation therapy, or infiltrative disorders, all of which cause secondary hypogonadism either by direct reduction in gonadotropin release or by producing hyperprolactinemia which reduces gonadotropin secretion and action. Men with chronic illness may develop hypothalamic hypogonadism. A number of drugs, hyperprolactinemia, hemochromatosis, and either endogenous or iatrogenic CS may also interfere with hypothalamic–pituitary–testicular function.

## CLINICAL PRESENTATION

The clinical presentation of male hypogonadism depends on the time of onset. If inadequate virilization occurs before the third month of intrauterine life, sexual ambiguity occurs. If it occurs during the third trimester, cryptorchidism and microphallus may result. Male hypogonadism in the postnatal prepubertal period results in failure of development of the phallus and scrotal rogation, as well as failure of development of secondary sexual characteristics (male voice, muscle mass, beard, and body hair), eunuchoidal proportions (due to failure of epiphyseal closure), and reduced bone mass.

Postpubertal hypogonadism results in diminished libido, erectile dysfunction, and variable degrees of reduction in male hair distribution. Bone density may be reduced and some men complain of a reduction in energy.

## DIAGNOSIS

Diagnosis is made by clinical examination (**188A–D**), as well as measurement of testosterone, gonadotropins and often genetic analysis (karyotype, **188E**). In the prepubertal male, evaluation of the external genitalia, testes, and somatic development will point to possible causes. In the postpuberal male, differentiation of testicular failure from secondary hypogonadism is critical, since detection of the latter should lead to a search for pituitary–hypothalamic disease, often a tumor. MRI of the pituitary–hypothalamic region is required in all cases of secondary hypogonadism.

Hypogonadotropic (secondary) hypogonadism is characterized by low levels of both testosterone and gonadotropins, while primary testicular failure exhibits high levels of FSH and LH. Since the former is primarily regulated by inhibin, seminiferous tubular dysfunction with normal Leydig cell function would show normal testerone and LH with high FSH levels and reduction in sperm counts.

## MANAGEMENT/TREATMENT

Androgen replacement may be accomplished with testosterone preparations administered either parenterally or transdermally. Oral replacement options carry a high risk of hepatic injury. Adequacy of dosing can be ascertained with serum testosterone levels. Excessive dosing can lead to polycythemia and venous thrombosis, as well as excessive prostate stimulation. Prostate size and PSA should be measured along with hematocrit and liver chemistries. Replacement testosterone may occasionally 'unmask' prostate cancer. Adequate replacement restores muscle and bone strength, as well as male beard and sexual behavior. In cases where hypogonadism is secondary to hyperprolactinemia or excessive steroids, correction of the underlying disorder will often result in a return to normal function.

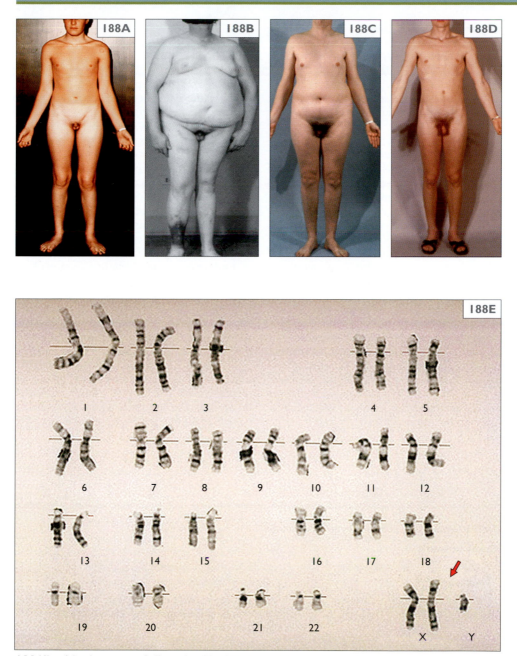

**188** Klinefelter's patients. **A**: Eunochoid body habitus, decreased pubic hair, gynecomastia; **B–D**: various presentations of hypogonadism; **E**: karyotype. (Courtesy of Dr. Donald Gordon.)

# Gynecomastia

## DEFINITION/OVERVIEW

Gynecomastia is a benign proliferation of male breast tissue. There is a trimodal age distribution with cases presenting during infancy, puberty, and adulthood.

## ETIOLOGY

Male breast tissue, like female breast tissue, is hormone responsive and demonstrates epithelial and ductal hyperplasia in response to estrogens. Therefore, in general, gynecomastia is caused by any process that increases the ratio of available estrogens compared to androgens (testosterone and androstendione). Sources of estrogen in the adult male include direct secretion by the testes (20%) and peripheral conversion of precursor hormones by aromatase in peripheral tissues (80%), mostly adipose tissue. Therefore increased estrogen levels can be due to over-secretion by source tissues, increased peripheral conversion to estradiol or estrone, or increased tissue sensitivity. Availability of estradiol is also increased by low sex-hormone binding globulin (SHBG) levels, because SHBG binds androgens with a higher affinity so that if SHBG levels are low, relatively more estrogen is available.

## PATHOGENESIS

Adolescents may develop a transient gynecomastia during puberty, most likely due to a brief imbalance between gonadal estrogen and androgen production. Most cases improve with time; however, some persist and account for about 25% of cases in adults.

In adults, the most common causes of gynecomastia include persistent pubertal gynecomastia (25%), medication-induced (10–25%), idiopathic (25%), cirrhosis (8%), and primary hypogonadism (8%). Drug-induced gynecomastia accounts for about 20% of cases (*Table 20*). Common culprits include spironolactone and finasteride.

Endocrine causes include hypogonadism (due to lower testosterone production but stable rates of peripheral conversion), obesity (due to increased peripheral conversion and decreased SHBG), and hyperprolactinemia (due to direct stimulation of breast tissue and secondary hypogonadism). Liver failure produces gynecomastia through multiple mechanisms including increased precursor formation by the adrenal gland, increased bioavailable estrone due to low albumin levels, decreased SHBG, and hypogonadism.

**Table 20 Mechanisms of drug-induced gynecomastia**

| Mechanism | drug |
| --- | --- |
| Increases estrogenic activity or increases estrogen production | Anabolic steroids, conjugated and synthetic estrogens, hCG, digoxin, clomiphene, phenytoin, diazepam |
| Decreases androgen activity or decreases androgen production | Ketoconazole, metronidazole, cimetidine, ranitidine, omeprazole, spironolactone, flutamide, methotrexate, isoniazid, penicillamine |
| Increases androgen clearance | Alcohol |
| Causes hyperprolactinemia | Metoclopramide, phenothiazine, haloperidol |
| Increases SHBG | Phenytoin, diazepam |

(Adapted from Ismail AA, JH Barth [2001]. *Annals of Clinical Biochemistry* **38**:596–607. Copyright 2001, RSM Press. All rights reserved.)

Hyperthyroidism, chronic renal insufficiency, smoking, and alchohol use are also associated with gynecomastia. Rare causes include testicular, adrenal, or hCG-producing germ cell tumors, and mild androgen insensitivity. Mild androgen insensitivity would present with gynecomastia, loss of sexual hair, and reduced fertility in association with increased LH and testosterone levels, with increased peripheral conversion of precursor hormones to estrogens.

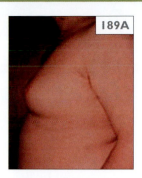

189 **A–C**: Bilateral gynecomastia. (Courtesy of gynecomastia.org.) **D**: Unilateral gynecomastia. (Courtesy of Dr. Donald Gordon.)

## CLINICAL PRESENTATION/ DIFFERENTIAL DIAGNOSIS

The differential diagnosis includes pseudo-gynecomastia (the presence of pendulous adipose tissue), benign soft tissue tumors (such as lipomas), and breast cancer. In true gynecomastia, glandular tissue can be felt as a palpable ridge that is symmetric and concentric to the nipple. It is usually bilateral, but can be unilateral (**189A–D**). Patients may also have breast pain. Breast cancer is usually unilateral, asymmetric to the nipple, and can be firm or fixed to underlying tissue. Skin changes and axillary lymphadenopathy may be present. Risk factors for breast cancer in men include Klinefelter's syndrome, orchitis, and cirrhosis. Imaging can be performed with ultrasound or mammography.

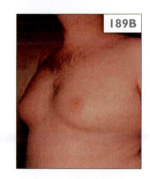

Examination should focus on the testicular examination and signs of systemic illness. Useful initial laboratory tests include testosterone, LH, SHBG, prolactin, and TSH levels. Estradiol levels can be measured in men but in most cases will not reveal the diagnosis. Serum hCG levels should be considered, especially if there is a history of rapid-onset breast enlargement or significant pain.

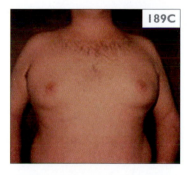

## TREATMENT

Pubertal gynecomastia usually regresses, but if symptoms persist or tissue exceeds 4 cm, an endocrine or medical diagnosis should be sought. In general, medications should be reviewed and treatment should be directed towards the underlying cause. However, if symptoms have been present for more than 2 years, it is likely that there is fibrosis of breast tissue and reduction mammoplasty may be required. The antiestrogen tamoxifen has also been used to treat gynecomastia and can be effective in some patients.

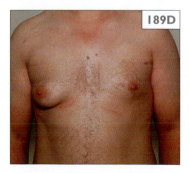

# Lipid disorders

Paraskevi Sapountzi

Norma Lopez

Francis Q. Almeda

**Lipid disorders**

**Lipoprotein (a)**

**Homocysteine**

**Future directions**

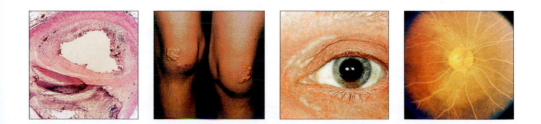

# Lipid disorders

## DEFINITION/OVERVIEW

Atherosclerotic cardiovascular disease (ASCVD) is the leading cause of mortality in the industrialized nations, and the cardiac event rates remain significant despite major advances in cardiovascular care. Abnormalities in lipid metabolism increase the risk for the development and progression of CHD and the diagnosis and treatment of patients with lipid disorders has been shown to significantly reduce the risk of future adverse cardiac events. In general, the intensity of risk reduction therapy should approximate the individual's absolute risk, and thus the accurate assessment of the patient's overall cardiovascular risk status is the central component for the optimal treatment of individuals with dyslipidemia.

The Executive Summary of the Third Report of the National Cholesterol Education Program (NCEP) Expert Panel on detection, evaluation, and treatment of high blood cholesterol in adults (Adult Treatment Panel III [ATP III]) provides evidence-based recommendations for the diagnosis and management of high cholesterol and related disorders in high-risk populations and primary prevention in patients with multiple risk factors. *Table 21* summarizes the definitions for elevated total cholesterol (TC), LDL, HDL, and triglycerides (TAGs).

## ETIOLOGY

Lipid disorders can be classified into primary (genetic or inherited) (see *Tables 23, 24*) or secondary (due to disease or environmental factors). Severe hypercholesterolemia (total cholesterol [TC] >350 mg/dL [>9 mmol/L]) has been associated with genetic abnormalities such as familial hypercholesterolemia with mutations in the LDL receptors, resulting in impaired clearance of LDL. Important secondary factors that result in altered lipid metabolism include hypothyroidism, diabetes mellitus, renal disease, obstructive liver disease, and alcohol intake. In addition, several medications such as estrogens/progestins, glucocorticoids, thiazides, isotretinoin, and cyclosporine have been associated with mild to moderate hypercholesterolemia.

**Table 21 ATP III lipid and lipoprotein classification**

**I. Total cholesterol mg/dL (mmol/L)**

| | | |
|---|---|---|
| <200 | (5.2) | Desirable |
| 200–239 | (5.2–6.2) | Borderline high |
| ≥240 | (6.2) | High |

**II. LDL cholesterol mg/dL (mmol/L)**

| | | |
|---|---|---|
| <100 | (2.6) | Optimal |
| 100–129 | (2.6–3.3) | Near optimal/above optimal |
| 130–159 | (3.4–4.1) | Borderline high |
| 160–189 | (4.2–4.9) | High |
| ≥190 | (5.0) | Very high |

**III. HDL cholesterol mg/dL (mmol/L)**

| | | |
|---|---|---|
| <40 (1.0) | (males) | Low |
| <50 (1.3) | (females) | |
| ≥60 (1.5) | | High |

**IV. Triglycerides (mg/dL)**

| | | |
|---|---|---|
| <150 | (1.6) | Normal |
| 150–199 | (1.6–2.1) | Borderline high |
| 200–499 | (2.2–5.4) | High |
| ≥500 | (5.5) | Very high |

## PATHOPHYSIOLOGY

The central concept of lipid transport is that plasma lipids circulate in lipoprotein particles. Lipoproteins are large complexes that transport lipids (mainly cholesterol esters, TAGs, and fat-soluble vitamins) between the vasculature and various body tissues. The plasma lipoproteins are divided into major classes based on their relative densities: chylomicrons, very low-density lipoproteins (VLDLs), intermediate-density lipoproteins (IDLs), LDLs, and HDLs and lipoprotein (a) (Lp(a)). There are 10 major human plasma apolipoproteins (*Table 22*).

Lipoprotein metabolism occurs through two basic mechanisms which include the transport of dietary lipids to the liver and peripheral tissues (exogenous pathway), and the production and delivery of hepatic lipids into the circulation and peripheral tissues (endogenous pathway). In the exogenous pathway, dietary cholesterol is acted upon by the intestinal cells to form cholesterol esters through the addition of fatty acids (**190**). TAGs from the diet are hydrolyzed by pancreatic lipases within the intestine and emulsified with bile acids to form micelles. Longer chain fatty acids are incorporated into TAGs and

**Table 22 Major human plasma apolipoproteins**

| Apolipoprotein | Major density class |
|---|---|
| A-I | HDL |
| A-II | HDL |
| A-IV | Chylomicrons, HDL |
| B-100 | VLDL, IDL, LDL |
| B-48 | Chylomicrons, VLDL, IDL |
| C-I | Chylomicrons, VLDL, IDL, HDL |
| C-II | Chylomicrons, VLDL, IDL, HDL |
| C-III | Chylomicrons, VLDL, IDL, HDL |
| E | Chylomicrons, VLDL, |
| Apo(a) | Lp(a)-density LDL to HDL |

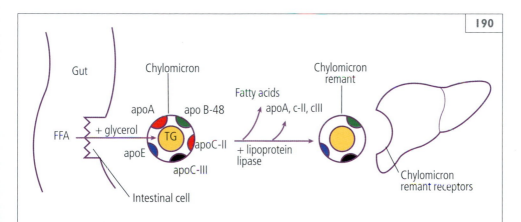

**190** Exogenous pathway of lipid metabolism. Free fatty acids are absorbed in the gastrointestinal tract and combine with glycerol in the intestinal cell to form triglycerides. These triglycerides combine with a variety of apolipoproteins including apo A, B-48, C-II, C-III, and E, the main one being apo B-48. This combination forms a very large particle called a chylomicron to carry the dietary lipid. The enzyme lipoprotein lipase hydrolyzes the core and releases fatty acids. The remnant is then taken up and cleared by the liver.

complexed with other particles such as cholesterol esters and phospholipids to form chylomicrons (which have a high concentration of TAG). These particles are acted upon by lipoprotein lipase along the capillary endothelium and the TAGs are hydrolyzed releasing free fatty acids, most of which are taken up by adjacent adipocytes or myocytes, and the remaining particles (chylomicron remnants) are transported to the liver.

In the endogenous pathway, VLDL is transformed into IDL and then into LDL through hepatic metabolism (**191**). VLDL particles are similar to chylomicrons, but have a higher ratio of cholesterol to TAG and contain apolipoprotein-B 100. The TAG of VLDL is hydrolyzed by lipoprotein lipase and the particles continue to become smaller and denser and transform into IDL, which is composed of similar amounts of cholesterol and TAG. The hepatic cells remove approximately half of VLDL remnants and IDL. The remainder of IDL is modified by hepatic lipase to form LDL. LDL is composed of a core of primarily cholesterol esters, surrounded by a surface of phospholipids, free cholesterol, and apolipoprotein B. The majority of circulating LDL is cleared through LDL-mediated endocytosis in the liver. Modified (oxidized) plasma LDL accumulates in the intima and is acted upon by activated macrophages (foam cells) and through complex mechanisms involving cytokines, growth factors, smooth cell proliferation, and inflammation and results in atheroma formation (**192**). The process of transferring cholesterol from peripheral cells to

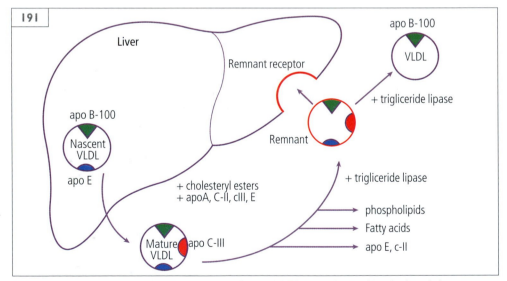

**191** Endogenous pathway of lipid metabolism. Nascent VLDL is synthesized by the liver. It becomes mature VLDL after addition of cholesterol esters and several apolipoproteins, the main ones as shown in the diagram. At this point lipoprotien lipase breaks down the VLDL into smaller remnants. The smaller VLDL remnants can then proceed down one of two paths: they can be taken up and cleared by the liver, or hydrolyzed and released as LDL.

the liver for removal from the body by biliary secretion is called reverse cholesterol transport. The role of HDL in enhancing reverse cholesterol transport is one of the mechanisms by which HDL protects against the process of atherosclerosis (**193**). The major protein of HDL is apo A-1.

## CLINICAL PRESENTATION

There are two kinds of genetic dyslipoproteinemia, which result in abnormal plasma levels of several classes of plasma lipoproteins: the hyperlipoproteinemias and the hypolipoproteinemias. The clinical presentation, physical exam, differential diagnosis, and laboratory evaluation of lipoproteinemias are summarized in *Tables 23* and *24* (*overleaf*). Important clinical

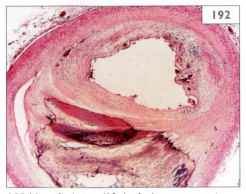

**192** Magnified view (10×) of atheroma seen in atherosclerosis. At this level, intima, media, and adventitia are evident. Blue areas in the media represent calcification. (Courtesy of J.H. Lim and C. Oyer, Brown University.)

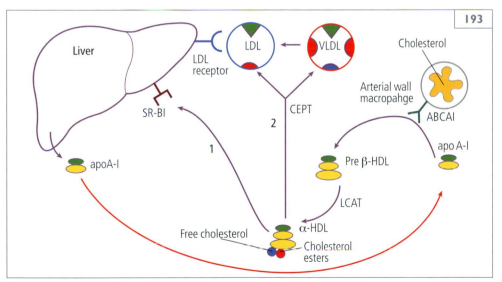

**193** HDL metabolism. The liver produces lipid-poor apolipoprotien A-I which removes excess cellular cholesterol by interacting with ABCAI. LCAT then esterifies this more lipid-rich particle into cholesterol esters which can either return to the liver directly to be taken up by SRB-1 (1) or they can transfer the cholesterol to VLDL and LDL (2). LDL can then be taken up by the liver via its receptor. ABCI: ATP-binding cassette transporter; CEPT: cholesterol ester transfer protein; HDL: high-density lipoprotein; LCAT: lecithin cholesterol acyltransferase; LDL: low-density lipoprotein; SRB-1: scavenger receptor class B, type 1; VLDL: very low-density lipoprotein.

Table 23 Clinical history, physical examination, and laboratory evaluation of hyperlipoproteinemias

| Hyperlipoproteinemia | Molecular defect | Lipoproteins | Major density class |
|---|---|---|---|
| Chylomicronemia syndrome | LPL (lipoprotein lipase) deficiency | ApoC-II deficiency | Chylomicrons elevated VLDL/IDL elevated |
| Familial hypercholesterolemia (FH) | Structural defect or absence of LDL receptor | Elevated plasma apoB | LDL elevated |
| Dysbetalipoproteinemia (Type III hyperlipoproteinemia) | Delayed clearance of remnants of TAG rich lipoproteins | ApoE deficiency | VLDL/IDL elevated |
| Familial combined hyperlipidemia (FCH) | To be established | Increased apoB-100 | LDL/VLDL elevated Often HDL reduced |
| Familial defective apoB-100 (FDB) | ApoB-100 mutation | Defective apoB-100 (the mutation affects the receptor binding domain of the protein decreasing the affinity of the mutant apoB-100 for its receptor to 3–5% of normal. The result is decreased receptor-mediated clearance of LDL from the circulation) | LDL elevated |

**Table 23 Clinical history, physical examination, and laboratory evaluation of hyperlipoproteinemias** (continued)

| Clinical history | Physical examination | Laboratory evaluation |
|---|---|---|
| Occurs in approximately 1 in a 1,000,000<br>Pancreatitis<br>Dry eyes & mouth<br>Numbness or tingling of the extremities<br>Neurophychiatric symptoms<br>  (depression & memory loss) | Eruptive xanthoma<br>Lipemic plasma<br>Lipemia retinalis<br>Hepatosplenomegaly | Very high TAG >1500 mg/dL<br>(15 mmol/L) |
| Occurs in 1 in 500<br>Premature CAD | Tendon xanthomas (in the dorsum<br>  of the hands and Achilles tendons)<br>Xanthomas<br>Xanthelasmas and xanthomas of<br>  the eyes<br>Arcus juvenilis | Heterozygous FH (LDL range<br>[325–450 mg/dL (8.5 –12 mmmol/L)]<br>Homozygous FH with very high LDL<br>[500–1000 mg/dL (13–26 mmol/L)]<br>Normal TAG |
| Premature CAD<br>Peripheral vascular disease | Palmar xanthomas (pathognomonic)<br>Tuberous xanthomas<br>Xanthelasma<br>Premature CAD | Elevated TC<br>Elevated TAG |
| Relatively common (up to 2% of<br>  population)<br>Premature CAD<br>Common comorbidity include diabetes,<br>  hypertension, and obesity | No tendon xanthomas<br>Xanthelasma<br>Arcus juvenilis<br>Eruptive xanthomas | Varying patterns of high LDL with<br>moderate elevations of TAG and low<br>HDL<br>LDL/apoB >1.3 (normal <1.3)<br>LDL/apoB >130 mg/dL (3.4 mmol/L) |
| Premature CAD | Arcus juvenilis<br>Tendon xanthomas<br>Xanthelasma | Elevated TC<br>Elevated LDL |

Table 24 Clinical history, physical examination, and laboratory evaluation of hypolipoproteinemias

| Hypolipoproteinemia | Molecular defect | Lipoproteins | Major density class |
|---|---|---|---|
| Tangier disease | ABCA1 transporter mutation | Decreased apoA-I | HDL <5 mg/dL 0.1 mmol/L) |
| Familial hypoalphalipo- proteinemia | ApoA-1 mutation | ApoA-1 deficiency ApoC-III deficiency ApoA-IV deficiency | LDL elevated |
| Abetalipoproteinemia (autosomal recessive) | Defect in assembly and secretion of apoB- containing lipoproteins | ApoB-100 deficiency ApoB-48 deficiency | Absence of ALDL/IDL, LDL |
| Familial hypobeta- lipoproteinemia | ApoB gene mutation | ApoB-48 and apoB-100 deficiency | Deficiency of chylomicrons and VLDL |
| Sitosterolemia | ABCG5 or ABCG8 mutation | Defective transporter (ABCG5 or ABCG8). This transporter preferentially transports plant and shellfish sterols from the intestine or liver into the gastrointestinal tract thus preventing absorption of the plant and shellfish sterols | Elevated plant and fish sterols |

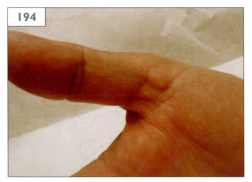

194 A 7 × 4 mm firm nodule representing a xanthomatous nodule of the flexor pollicis brevis in a patient with hypercholesterolemia. (Courtesy of foto@finlay-online.org.)

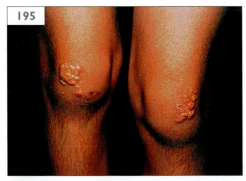

195 Cutaneous xanthomas in homozygous familial hypercholesterolemia. (From Teruel JL, Lasunción MA. Images in clinical medicine. Cutaneous xanthoma in homozygous familial hypercholesterolemia. *N Engl J Med* 1995:**332**(17):1137. Copyright 1995 Massachusetts Medical Society. All rights reserved.)

**Table 24** Clinical history, physical examination, and laboratory evaluation of hypolipoproteinemias (continued)

| Clinical history | Physical examination | Laboratory evaluation |
|---|---|---|
| Modest increased risk of premature CAD | Orange-yellow tonsils (pathognomonic) Corneal opacities Peripheral neuropathy | TC1 < 120 mg/dL (3.1 mmol/L) Normal or elevated TAG |
| Most common genetic cause of low HDL. HDL below 10th percentile with normal cholesterol and TAG levels after secondary causes of low HDL excluded Premature CAD | Often associated with obesity, metabolic syndrome, diabetes | Low HDL |
| Steatorrhea Cardiac arrythmias | Neurologic dysfunction Nystagmus Retinitis pigmentosa Progressive blindness | TC <50 mg/dL (13 mmol/L) Low TAG Vitamin A and E deficiency Hemolytic anemia (acanthocytes) |
| Mild malabsorption | Absence of neurologic dysfunction Progressive degeneration | Mild deficiency of fat-soluble vitamins |
| Premature CAD Arthralgias Arthritis at a young age | Tendon xanthomas Tuberous xanthomas Hypersplenism | Elevated TC Elevated plant and fish sterols [500–600 mg/dL (13–15.6 mmol/L)] Hemolytic anemia |

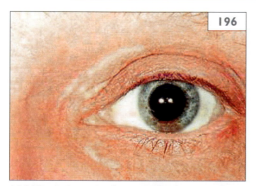

**196** Xanthelasma in the periorbital region of a patient with hypercholesterolemia. (Reprinted from Dorlands Dictionary 30th edn. Copyright 2004, with permission from Elsevier.)

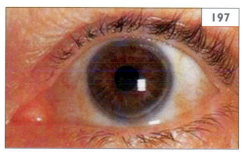

**197** Arcus juvenilis is an opaque circle around the cornea, identical to arcus senilis but occurring in young people. Deposits of lipids cause a white ring around the periphery of the cornea and when seen in a young person it can be associated with hypercholesterolemia. (Courtesy of www.argy-bargey.blogspot.com.)

findings in patients with significant hypercholesterolemia include xanthomas (**194, 195**), xanthelasma (**196**), arcus juvenilis (**197**), and lipid keratopathy (**198**). The chylomicronemia syndrome results in very high triglyceride levels of >1500 mg/dL (15 mmol/L) and is associated with eruptive xanthoma (**199, 200**), a creamy layer on top of plasma left overnight in a refrigerator (**201**), and lipemia retinalis (**202**). Palmar xanthomas (**203**) are often demonstrated in patients with dysbetalipoproteinemia.

Elevated LDL, low HDL, and elevated TAG are associated with progressive atherosclerosis in

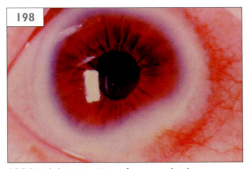

198

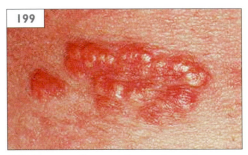

199

198 Lipid degeneration of cornea also known as lipid keratopathy appears as a dense yellow-cream colored opacification or cholesterol crystals on the corneal stroma surrounding blood vessels as a result of cholesterol or free fatty acid infiltration. The primary form is often bilateral and can occur in conditions such as Tangiers disease. (Courtesy of www.eyeatlas.com.)

199 Close up of an eruptive xanthoma in a patient with hypercholesterolemia. (Reprinted from Dorlands Dictionary 30th edn. Copyright 2004, with permission from Elsevier.)

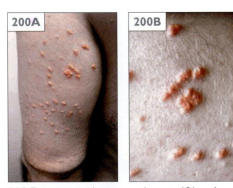

200A 200B

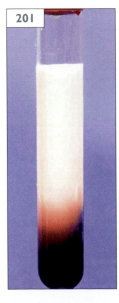

201

200 Eruptive xanthomas on the arm (**A**) and upper torso (**B**) in a patient with severe hypertriglyceridemia. (From Nayak KR, Daly RG. Images in clinical medicine. Eruptive xanthomas associated with hypertriglyceridemia and new-onset diabetes mellitus. *N Engl J Med* 2004:**350**(12)1235. Copyright 2004 Massachusetts Medical Society. All rights reserved.)

201 Creamy layer on top of plasma left overnight in a refrigerator, usually occurs when triglycerides are over 1500mg/dL. (From Fred HL, Accad M. Images in clinical medicine. Lipemia retinalis. *N Engl J Med* 1999:**340**(25):1969. Copyright 1999 Massachusetts Medical Society. All rights reserved.)

the coronary, carotid, cerebral, and peripheral vasculature (**204**). Acute MI often occurs in coronary plaques with 'mild' stenoses (<50%), and factors associated with plaque rupture include a large lipid core, thin fibrous cap, and activated macrophages, inflammatory cytokines. Rupture often occurs at the lateral edge or 'shoulder' at the interface of plaque and normal intima. Acute MI usually occurs when a 'vulnerable' atherosclerotic plaque ruptures with subsequent thrombosis and occlusion of coronary flow (**205**), and is treated with either thrombolytic therapy or percutaneous coronary intervention. Cholesterol emboli syndrome may

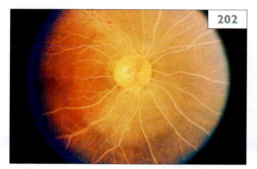

**202** Lipemia retinalis, characterized by the creamy white appearance of retinal vessels, is a funduscopic finding occuring with very high triglyceride levels that can be seen in chylomicronemia syndrome. (From Fred HL, Accad M. Images in clinical medicine. Lipemia retinalis. *N Engl J Med* 1999: **340**(25):1969. Copyright 1999 Massachusetts Medical Society. All rights reserved.)

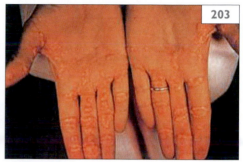

**203** Palmar xanthomas are pathognomonic for dysbetalipoproteinemia-Type III. (Courtesy of Dr. Pham Thi Thu Thuy.)

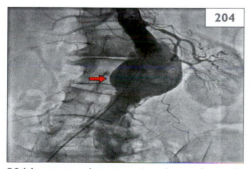

**204** Aortogram demonstrating a large infrarenal abdominal aortic aneurysm measuring approximately 6.0 cm (arrow) with an associated severe stenosis of the proximal left renal artery

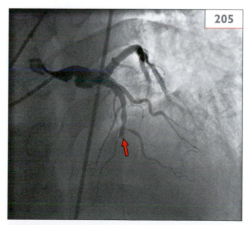

**205** Coronary angiogram in a patient who presented with chest pain and an acute ST segment elevation myocardial infarction, demonstrating a large thrombus totally occluding the mid left anterior descending artery (arrow).

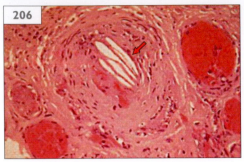

206 Characteristic needle-shaped clefts (arrow) resulting from atheroemboli. (From Bradley M. Images in clinical medicine. Spontaneous atheroembolism. *N Engl J Med* 1995:**332**(15):998. Copyright 1995 Massachusetts Medical Society. All rights reserved.)

occur after any invasive arterial procedure, and although may also occur spontaneously. The clinical syndrome may involve worsening renal function, hypertension, and distal ischemia and may be associated with characteristic dermatologic and ophthalmologic findings (206–208). The pathophysiology of this syndrome may involve cholesterol crystals showering the distal vascular beds with the associated local vasospastic mediators, or larger cholesterol plaques breaking off and occluding the peripheral vessels resulting in tissue and organ ischemia.

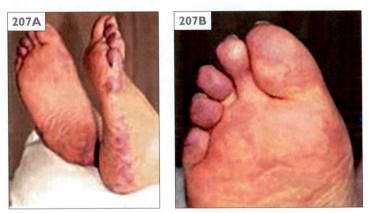

207 Cholesterol emboli demonstrated by livedo reticularis on the legs and a bluish discoloration of the toes in a patient 12 hours after a cardiac catheterization. (From xx. xxxx. *N Engl J Med* 2006;**352**(12):1294. Copyright 2006 Massachusetts Medical Society. All rights reserved.)

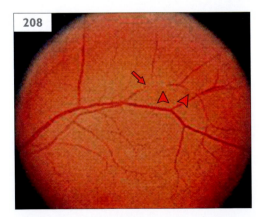

208 Fundoscopic examination showing a cholesterol emboli (arrow) at the bifurcation of a retinal and vascular sheathing distal to the occlusion (arrowheads). (From Bradley M. Images in clinical medicine. Spontaneous atheroembolism. *N Engl J Med* 1995;**332**(15):998. Copyright 1995 Massachusetts Medical Society. All rights reserved.)

## DIFFERENTIAL DIAGNOSIS

The diagnosis of elevated lipoproteins can be established with the appropriate laboratory tests. If an underlying genetic abnormality is present, the diagnosis is suggested by the severity and pattern of the lipoprotein abnormalities, the family history, and the presence of premature atherosclerotic vascular disease. The history, physical examination and laboratory evaluation remain crucial for the proper diagnosis as well as the appropriate treatment (*Tables 23, 24*). Certain clinical features such as tendon xanthomas help distinguish familial hypercholesterolemia (present) from familial combined hypercholesterolemia (absent) (**209A, B, 210**). Some of the rare entities have pathognomonic or characteristic clinical findings, such as orange-yellow tonsils in

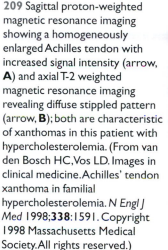
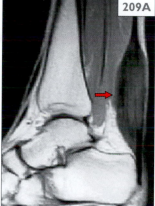
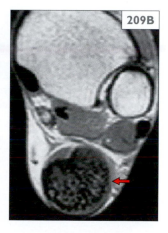

**209** Sagittal proton-weighted magnetic resonance imaging showing a homogeneously enlarged Achilles tendon with increased signal intensity (arrow, **A**) and axial T-2 weighted magnetic resonance imaging revealing diffuse stippled pattern (arrow, **B**); both are characteristic of xanthomas in this patient with hypercholesterolemia. (From van den Bosch HC, Vos LD. Images in clinical medicine. Achilles' tendon xanthoma in familial hypercholesterolemia. *N Engl J Med* 1998;**338**:1591. Copyright 1998 Massachusetts Medical Society. All rights reserved.)

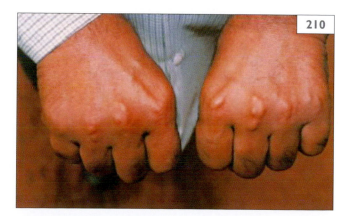

**210** Tendon xanthomas in a patient with hypercholesterolemia. (From *JIACM* 2003;**4**(1):69, with permission.)

Tangier disease (**211, 212**). It is essential to rule out secondary factors that result in altered lipid metabolism including hypothyroidism, diabetes mellitus, renal disease, obstructive liver disease, and alcohol intake, and medications such as estrogens/progestins, glucocorticoids, thiazides, and cyclosporine.

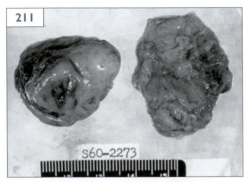

**211** Enlarged tonsils seen in Tangier disease. (Courtesy of the National Institutes of Health.)

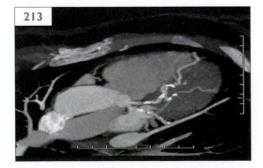

**212** Enlarged orange-yellow tonsils in a patient with Tangier disease.

## DIAGNOSIS

The diagnosis of hypercholesterolemia is established by laboratory data and supported by comprehensive history and physical exam. LDL subclasses may be measured through nuclear magnetic resonance spectroscopy, and the detection of smaller denser LDL particles may provide incremental information on cardiovascular risk.

Significant dyslipidemia often results in progressive cardiovascular disease, and various imaging modalities for measuring clinical and subclinical atherosclerotic vascular disease include exercise and chemical stress testing, arterial Doppler evaluation, MRI, and conventional coronary and peripheral angiography. The availability of newer technology such as cardiac CT (64-slice and above) provides an excellent noninvasive tool for the evaluation of degree and extent of coronary plaque (**213**).

## MANAGEMENT/TREATMENT

The largest body of evidence exists for improved outcomes with LDL lowering, and thus LDL remains the major therapeutic target for intervention. Large epidemiologic studies have confirmed the continuous and graded association of total serum cholesterol and coronary heart disease. Large, placebo controlled, randomized trials have confirmed the benefit of LDL lowering on reducing long-term cardiac event rates in both primary and secondary prevention. Although LDL remains the primary lipid lowering priority, a low HDL and high TAG have been associated with increased cardiac risk and are potential targets for therapeutic intervention. Pooled data from several studies estimate a 2–3% reduction in

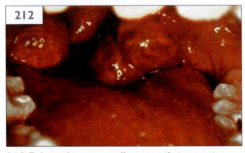

**213** Coronary angiogram using a 64-slice computed tomography, demonstrating severe atherosclerosis with multiple mixed calcified and soft plaque in the left anterior descending artery and circumflex artery.

cardiovascular risk for every 1 mg/dL increase in HDL. If the TAG level is ≥500 mg/dL (5.6 mmol/L), then treatment of TAG takes priority over LDL reduction due to the desire to lower the risk of acute pancreatitis.

The central principle of management of the patient with dyslipidemia is that the intensity of risk reduction should be commensurate with the individual's absolute cardiovascular risk (*Table 25*). The major risk factors (exclusive of LDL cholesterol) include age ≥45 years in men and ≥55 years in women, cigarette smoking, hypertension (defined as ≥140/90 mmHg or on antihypertensive medication), low HDL cholesterol (<40 mg/dL [1 mmol/L]), family history of premature coronary heart disease in a first degree relative (<55 years in male relative, and <65 years in female relative). The 10-year risk of a cardiac event is assessed by using the Framingham scoring which takes into account these factors, and may be calculated using tables or handheld and internet-based online

**Table 25 LDL-cholesterol goals and cutpoints for therapeutic lifestyle changes (TLC) and drug therapy in different risk categories**

| Risk category | LDL goal mg/dL (mmol/L) | LDL level at which to initiate TLC mg/dL (mmol/L) | LDL level at which to consider drug therapy mg/dL (mmol/L) |
|---|---|---|---|
| CHD* or CHD risk equivalents (10-year risk >20%) | <100 (2.6) | ≥100++ (2.6) | ≥130 (3.3) <br> 100–129 (2.6–3.3): drug optional <br> <100 (2.6) in selected high risk populations+ |
| 2+ Risk factors** (10-year risk ≤20%) | <130 (3.4) | ≥130 (3.4) | 10-year risk 10–20% <br> ≥130 (3.4)# <br> 10-year risk <10% <br> ≥160 (4.1) |
| 0–1 Risk factor | <160 (4.1) | ≥160 (4.1) | ≥190 (4.9) <br> 160–189 (4.1-4.9): LDL-lowering drug optional |

(Courtesy of the National Heart, Lung, and Blood Institute.)

*CHD includes established coronary artery disease (history of myocardial infarction, unstable or stable angina, coronary revascularization, or evidence of clinically significant myocardial ischemia). CHD equivalents include diabetes and evidence of noncoronary atherosclerosis (peripheral arterial disease, abdominal aortic aneurysm, carotid artery disease, transient ischemic attacks, or stroke).

**Risk factors include: age (men >45 years and women >55 years), hypertension (BP >140/90 mmHg or on antihypertensive medication), smoking, low HDL (<40 mg/dL [1 mmol/L]), and family history of premature CAD (CHD in male first degree relative <55 years; CHD in female first degree relative <65 years).

+Very high risk favors the optional LDL-C goal of 70 mg/dL (1.8 mmol/L), and in patients with high triglycerides and low HDL.

++In individual at high risk or moderately high risk with lifestyle-related risk factors (i.e. obesity, physical inactivity, elevated triglycerides, low HDL, metabolic syndrome), aggressive therapeutic lifestyle changes to modify these risk factors is advisable regardless of the LDL level.

#For moderately high-risk individuals, if the LDL is 100–129 mg/dL (2.6–3.3 mmol/L) at baseline or on TLC, initiation of an LDL-lowering drug to achieve an LDL of <100 mg/dL (2.6 mmol/L) is a therapeutic option.

calculators (www.nhlbi.nih.gov/guidelines/cholesterol). The highest risk group includes those patients with established cardiovascular disease or a 'CHD risk equivalent'. This group is comprised of patients with known coronary artery disease, other clinical forms of atherosclerotic vascular disease including peripheral vascular disease, carotid artery disease, abdominal aortic aneurysm, and diabetes mellitus, and patients with multiple risk factors that confer a risk for a major cardiac event of >20% over 10 years. The identification of subclinical atherosclerotic disease such as high coronary calcification, significant carotid intimal medial thickness, or significant atherosclerotic burden on CT angiography likewise warrants aggressive and intensive lipid lowering.

Recent trials have demonstrated incremental reductions in risk for adverse cardiac events with LDL levels lowered to below 100 mg/dL (2.6 mmol/L). Overall, these data suggest that there is no clear-cut identifiable threshold for LDL level for risk reduction and that 'lower is better'. Based on these new trials demonstrating reduced cardiovascular event rates with lower LDL levels, the current recommendation for optimal LDL is <70 mg/dL (1.8 mmol/L) in patients with the highest risk, including those with established ASCVD and CHD equivalents, and multiple major risk factors. No major safety issues have been identified thus far with lowering LDL in the range of 50–70 mg/dL (1.3–1.8 mmol/L).

## Therapeutic modalities for dyslipidemia

A summary of the available agents for hypercholesterolemia is provided in *Table 26*.

### Dietary modification

Lifestyle and dietary modification remain the cornerstone of therapy and reduced intake of saturated fat and cholesterol, increased physical activity, and weight control for all patients is strongly recommended. All patients should be advised to adopt therapeutic lifestyle changes (TLCs) including reduced intake of saturated fats (<7% of total calories) and cholesterol (<200 mg/d), increased intake of soluble fiber (10–25 g/day), weight reduction, and increased physical activity. However, although dietary modification should be a mainstay of any LDL lowering strategy, the average LDL reduction from diet alone is in the range of 5–10%. HDL levels have been shown to increase with weight reduction, regular aerobic exercise, modest alcohol consumption, and smoking cessation. Typically, one may expect a 1 mg/dL increase in HDL for every 3 kg weight loss. Regular aerobic exercise may increase HDL by 10–20% in sedentary adults.

### Statins (3-hydroxy-3-methylglutaryl coenzyme A reductase inhibitors)

Statins lower serum LDL levels through intracellular inhibition of the rate-limiting step in cholesterol production, which reduces cholesterol biosynthesis in the liver and upregulates LDL receptors to increase clearance of LDL from the blood. The statins lower the LDL by 18–55%, increase HDL by 5–15%, and lower TAG by 7–30% (*Table 21*). At the current available doses, rosuvastatin and atorvastatin are the most potent statins followed in order of LDL lowering potency by simvastatin, lovastatin, pravastatin, and fluvastatin. Each doubling of a statin dose achieves an approximately 6% additional reduction in serum LDL (the 'rule of 6s'). A large meta-analysis involving 14 randomized, placebo-controlled trials involving 90,056 patients showed that lowering LDL-cholesterol levels by 39 mg/dL (1 mmol/L) with statin therapy significantly reduces the 5-year risk of major coronary events, coronary revascularization, and stroke by 21%. Although treatment with statins has resulted in major reductions in cardiac event rates, the amount of plaque regression demonstrated has been modest at most, raising the possibility that the beneficial effects extend over and beyond LDL lowering, including anti-inflammatory, antithrombotic, immunomodulatory, and vascular effects.

Statins are generally well-tolerated; however, common minor side-effects include muscle and joint aches (up to 5%), fatigue, dyspepsia, and headaches. More serious side-effects such as severe myositis with generalized muscle pain and weakness and elevated creatine kinase (rarely leading to rhabdomyolysis and acute renal failure) or severe hepatitis may occur infrequently. Adverse drug interactions should be carefully monitored, particularly at higher doses and in elderly patients with low body weight, and in patients with impaired renal function or on combination therapy with fibrates and/or nicotinic acid.

**Table 26 Drugs for treating lipoprotein abnormalities**

| Drugs | Lipid effects | Adverse effects/drug interactions |
|---|---|---|
| **Statins** | | |
| Pravastatin (40–80 mg at bedtime) Lovastatin (2 –80 mg at bedtime) Fluvastatin (20–80 mg at bedtime) Simvastatin (20–80mg at bedtime) Atorvostatin (10–80 mg at bedtime) transaminase Rosuvastatin (10–40 mg at bedtime) | LDL: ⇓18–55% HDL: ⇑5–15% TAG: ⇓7–30% | Increased risk of myopathy with itraconazole, ketoconazole, erythromycin, clarithromycin, HIV protease inhibitors, nefazodone, amiodarone, verapamil, or large quantities of grapefruit juice (>1 quart [<1L] daily); may raise hepatic levels |
| **Cholesterol absorption inhibitor** | | |
| Ezetimibe (10 mg daily) | LDL: ⇓ 15–20% HDL: ⇑ 2–5% TAG: ⇓ 3–8% | Side-effects include headache and diarrhea; myopathy and hepatitis rare |
| **Fibric acids** | | |
| Gemfibrozil (600 mg twice per day) Fenofibrate (48–145 mg or 43–130 mg daily) | LDL: ⇓5–20% HDL: ⇑ 10–20% TAG: ⇓ 20–55% | Side-effects include rash and dyspepsia; potentiates the action of warfarin; contraindicated in patients with gallstones, or severe renal insufficiency/ hemodialysis; variable effects on serum LDL, and may increase LDL |
| **Nicotinic acids** | | |
| Immediate-release (100 mg–2 g 3 times daily) Sustained-release (250 mg–1.5 g twice daily) Extended-release (500 mg–2 g at bedtime) | LDL: ⇓ 5–20% HDL: ⇑ 15–35% TAG: ⇓ 20–50% | Most common side-effect is flushing; potentiates the action of warfarin; may precipitate acute gout and esophageal reflux, hyperglycemia |
| **Bile acid sequestrants** | | |
| Cholestryramine (4–24 g/day) Colestipol (5–40 g/day) Colesevelam (3750–4375 mg daily) | LDL: ⇓ 15–30% HDL: ⇑ 3–5% TAG: ⇑ 3–10% | Common side-effects include nausea, constipation and bloating; associated with increased TAG levels |
| **Fish oils** | | |
| Omega 3 fatty acid (3–12 g) | LDL: ⇑ 45% HDL: ⇑ 9% TAG: ⇓ 45% | Associated with increased LDL level; side-effects include dyspepsia and fishy aftertaste |

## Ezetimibe (cholesterol absorption inhibitor)

Ezetimibe acts through inhibition of intestinal cholesterol absorption in the small intestine leading to a reduction in hepatic cholesterol stores, increasing clearance of cholesterol from the blood. As monotherapy, ezetimibe effectively decrease LDL by 15–20%. The combination of ezetimibe and a statin provides a dual effect by inhibiting cholesterol intestinal absorption and cholesterol production in the liver, respectively. This combination lowers the LDL by as much as an additional 25%, with potentially fewer side-effects. Large randomized clinical trials evaluating the effect of the combination of ezetimibe and simvastatin compared with simvastin alone on 'hard' clinical end-points such as mortality and MI are currently underway.

## Bile acid sequestrants (resins)

Bile acid sequestrants act through binding bile acids in the intestine resulting in increased excretion in the stool, stimulating greater intrahepatic cholesterol utilization for bile acid synthesis. This results in upregulation of the LDL receptor, which enhances clearance of LDL in the bloodstream. In general, resins lower LDL by 15–30%. The available bile acid sequestrants include cholestryramine, colesevelam, and colestipol. Treatment with cholestyramine has been associated with a reduction in progression of atherosclerosis compared to control. Since resins are not systemically absorbed, they are extremely safe; however, they are associated with side-effects such as nausea, constipation, and bloating. Other medications should be taken either 1 hour before or 4 hours after the resins due to binding and decreased absorption (i.e. warfarin, digoxin). Resins may significantly raise the TAG level and should be avoided in patients with hypertriglyceridemia.

## Nicotinic acid

Nicotinic acid, or niacin, is a B-complex vitamin that raises HDL by 15–35%, decreases TAG by 20–50%, and modestly lowers LDL (approximately 5–20%). Niacin raises HDL through metabolic pathways that increase the pre-B, apoA-I rich HDL particles, which is the cardioprotective subfraction of HDL. Treatment with niacin reduced the risk of nonfatal MI even after 15 years of follow-up. The most common side-effect is cutaneous flushing, and the major adverse side-effect is hepatoxicity.

## Fibric acids

Fibrates are agonists of PPARα, which is a nuclear receptor involved in the modulation of lipid and carbohydrate metabolism. Fibrates increase hydrolysis of TAG by enhancing lipoprotein lipase activity, increasing clearance of TAG rich lipoproteins from the plasma, and decreasing the rate of release of free fatty acids from adipocytes. Fibrates are the most effective agents for reducing TAG (20–55%), and also effectively raise HDL (10–20%). These agents have variable effects on the serum LDL, and treated patients with hypertriglyceridemia may have an increase in their LDL. Fibrates are the drug of choice in patients with severe hypertriglyceridemia (>1000 mg/dL [11 mmol/L]). These drugs have been shown to be beneficial in both primary prevention and in patients with established coronary artery disease.

## Fish oils

Fish oils contain a high concentration of polyunsaturated fatty acids, and have been shown to reduce plasma triglycerides significantly, up to 45%, although they may be associated with increased LDL levels. Omega-3-acid ethyl esters are available as an adjunct to diet for the reduction of very high TAG levels (≥500 mg/dL [5.5 mmol/L]) in adults. The mechanism of action is poorly defined but may involve the inhibition of acyl Coa:1,2-diacylglycerol acyltransferase and increased peroxisomal β-oxidation in the liver.

## Nonpharmacologic strategies for lowering LDL-cholesterol

LDL apheresis involves the direct removal of LDL from the plasma and may be the preferred option in severe drug-resistant or refractory hyperlipidemia. Partial ileal bypass surgically depletes the enterohepatic supply of bile acids resulting in upregulation of the LDL receptor in the liver increasing LDL clearance, and may be an option in patients with severely elevated LDL and normal TAG refractory to maximal medical management who are not candidates for LDL apheresis.

## New treatment options for raising HDL

Cholesterol ester transfer protein (CETP) is a plasma glycoprotein produced in the liver that circulates in the bloodstream bound to HDL, that facilitates transfer of cholesterol esters between lipoproteins. CETP inhibition is a potential new therapy. CETP activity is potentially atherogenic and results in the net transfer of cholesterol esters from HDL to VLDL and LDL, thereby decreasing the concentration of HDL and increasing the concentration of LDL. Pharmacologically inhibiting CETP has been shown to increase the reverse cholesterol transport to the liver by increasing HDL and enhancing the hepatic uptake of cholesterol via scavenger receptor B-1 (SRB-1). However, CETP inhibition with torcetrapib was associated with increased mortality in a phase III clinical trial diminishing the enthusiasm for this class of drugs.

Other novel therapies under investigation for raising HDL include direct infusions of plasma-derived or synthetic apolipoprotein A-1, and agents that augment the expression of scavenger receptors.

## Lipoprotein (a)

Lipoprotein (a) (Lp(a)) is a lipoprotein similar to LDL in lipid and protein concentration, but is composed of two protein particles, apolipo-protein (Apo) B-100 and apolipoprotein (a). The precise role of Lp(a) in the pathogenesis and progression of atherosclerosis remains controversial, but potential mechanisms of Lp(a) include binding to proinflammatory oxidized phospholipids, decreased nitric oxide synthesis, increased leukocyte adhesion and smooth muscle proliferation, and inhibition of the fibrinolytic system. However, there remains substantial uncertainty regarding the role of Lp(a) in clinical practice, although an elevated level might warrant more aggressive treatment in patients who have high-risk family histories but few other risk factors. Statins do not decrease Lp(a) levels. Niacin is currently the only available lipid-lowering drug that significantly reduces the plasma levels of Lp(a).

## Homocysteine

An elevated level of homocysteine has been implicated as a risk factor for coronary athero-sclerosis, although the precise pathophysiology behind this association remains undefined. Treatment of hyperhomocysteinemia with folic acid and vitamin $B_6$ has shown mixed results in terms of lowering subsequent cardiac events. Recent data from large randomized clinical trials have demonstrated that the combination of high-dose vitamin B6 and folic acid lowered homocysteine levels by approximately 28%, but was associated with an increased risk of stroke and MI.

## Future directions

The optimal diagnostic and therapeutic approach to lipid disorders remains a crucial component of contemporary clinical practice. The increasing prevalence of obesity, metabolic syndrome, and diabetes mellitus continue to fuel the need for comprehensive treatment strategies for dealing with multiple lipid and metabolic disorders. LDL-cholesterol will remain the primary target for intervention; however, new treatment options for raising HDL cholesterol and lowering TAGs will continue to evolve rapidly. The proper identification and assessment of the patients at increased risk for the development and progression of atherosclerotic cardiovascular disease, and the selection of the appropriate goals for therapy will continue to be the main focus of basic science research and clinical trials in the future.

# Multiple endocrine neoplasia, neuroendocrine tumors, and other endocrine disorders

Teck-Kim Khoo

Mihaela Cosma

Hossein Gharib

**Multiple endocrine neoplasia type 1**

**Multiple endocrine neoplasia type 2**

**Carcinoid syndrome**

**Autoimmune polyglandular syndromes**

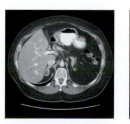
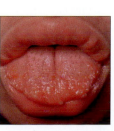
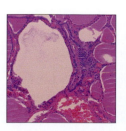
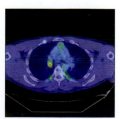

# Multiple endocrine neoplasia type 1

## DEFINITION/OVERVIEW
Multiple endocrine neoplasia type 1 (MEN1) is a rare clinical syndrome defined by having two out of the three main tumors: parathyroid, pituitary, and entero-pancreatic (*Table 27*).

However, over 20 endocrine and nonendocrine tumors can be seen in this syndrome. The prevalence of the disease is 2 in 100 000. When the index patient with MEN1 has a first degree relative with one of the three tumors, this is considered to be familial MEN1.

## ETIOLOGY/PATHOPHYSIOLOGY
This syndrome is inherited in an autosomal dominant manner (**214**) and is due to a mutation in the MEN1 gene which is located in the long arm of chromosome 11 (11q13). This mutation causes disruption of a 610-amino acid protein, menin. The exact role of menin and the mechanism by which this leads to MEN1 are still unclear, but is thought to be a loss of tumor suppressor function. This conveys an autosomal dominant predisposition to neoplasia in certain tissues.

## CLINICAL PRESENTATION
### Parathyroid
Primary hyperparathyroidism (PHP) is the most common manifestation, occurring in almost all patients by the age of 50. Unlike sporadic hyperparathyroidism, both genders are equally affected. MEN1 patients often present at a younger age than sporadic hyperparathyroidism, usually in their twenties. The signs and symptoms are similar to those of sporadic hyperparathyroidism, including asymptomatic or symptomatic hypercalcemia and osteoporosis. Symptoms of hypercalcemia may include constipation, nephrolithiasis, and neuropsychiatric manifestations, while osteoporosis may present as fractures. MEN1 typically involves multiple parathyroid glands (**215**).

### Entero-pancreatic
The presence of entero-pancreatic tumors is the second most common manifestation of MEN1, with gastrinomas being the most frequent. About 40% of MEN1 patients have gastrinomas, usually occurring in the duodenum, while 25% of patients with gastrinomas have MEN1. These patients may present with multiple recurrent peptic ulcers (**214**). Other tumors may secrete insulin, somatostatin, VIP or pancreatic polypeptide, although these may not always

---

**Table 27 Expression of MEN 1 with estimated penetrance by age 40**

Endocrine features Nonendocrine features

Parathyroid adenoma (90%) Lipoma (30%)

Entero-pancreatic tumor Facial angiofibroma (85%)

- **Gastrinoma** (40%) Collagenoma (70%)
- Insulinoma (10%)
- **NF** including pancreatic polypeptide (20%[a]) Rare, maybe innate, endocrine, or nonendocrine features
- Other: **glucagonoma, VIPoma, somatostatinoma** etc. (2%)

Foregut carcinoid

- **Thymic carcinoid** NF (2%) Pheochromocytoma (<1%)
- **Bronchial carcinoid** NF (2%) Ependymoma (1%)
- Gastric enterochromaffin-like tumor NF (10%)

Anterior pituitary tumor

- Prolactinoma (20%)
- Other: GH + PRL, GH, NF (each 5%)
- ACTH (2%), TSH (rare)

Adrenal cortex NF (25%)

**Bold** indicates tumor type with substantial (>25% of that tumor type) malignant potential. NF: Nonfunctioning. May synthesize a peptide hormone or other factors (such as small amine) but does not usually oversecrete enough to produce hormonal expression; a: omits nearly 100% prevalence of NF and clinically silent tumors, some of which are detected incidental to pancreatic-duodenal surgery in MEN1. ACTH: adrenocorticotrophic hormone; GH: growth hormone; PRL: prolactin; TSH: thyroid-stimulating hormone.

(Reprinted from Brandi ML, *et al.* Guidelines for diagnosis and therapy of MEN type I and type 2. *J Clin Endocrinol Metab* 2001;**86**:5658–71. Copyright 2001, The Endocrine Society, with permission.)

have clinical significance. Occasionally, islet cell tumors can be cystic. Entero-pancreatic tumors have a high metastatic potential, with almost half having spread to regional lymph nodes or the liver at diagnosis.

## Pituitary

Pituitary tumors occur in about 20–42% of MEN patients. Up to three-quarters of these are prolactinomas, although GH and ACTH can also be secreted. About 5% are non-functional. Clinical manifestations, therefore, are related to the type of hormone secreted. Pituitary tumors appear to be larger in size in MEN1 patients compared to those without the syndrome.

About one-third of MEN1 patients also have adrenocortical lesions (**216**). These are usually bilateral, nonfunctional hyperplasia although hyperaldosteronism, CS, pheochromocytoma, and adrenocortical carcinoma have been reported. Many also demonstrate visceral and cutaneous lipomas and angio-fibromas. Carcinoids of the foregut, thymus, or bronchial tree can also be found in association with MEN1.

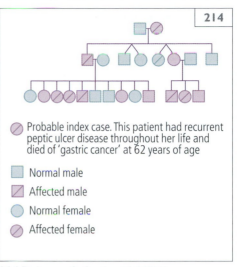

⊘ Probable index case. This patient had recurrent peptic ulcer disease throughout her life and died of 'gastric cancer' at 62 years of age

☐ Normal male

▨ Affected male

◯ Normal female

⊘ Affected female

**214** Pedigree of a family with MEN1.

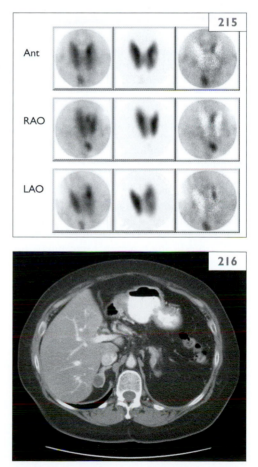

**215** Parathyroid Tc$^{99m}$ sestamibi of MEN1 patient with left superior and right inferior parathyroid adenomas, demonstrating multiple areas of discordant uptake.

Ant

RAO

LAO

**216** Bilateral adrenal enlargement. There is a 1.9 cm homogenous mass of decreased attenuation in the right adrenal gland suggestive of an adenoma, while the left adrenal gland (seen best on another view) is homogenously enlarged as well, measuring 1.4 cm in its maximal view. Noted as well is the distal pancreatectomy, splenectomy.

## DIFFERENTIAL DIAGNOSIS

More frequently, these endocrinopathies occur sporadically and more than one may be present in a single patient without MEN1. A positive family history or multiple parathyroid hyperplasia should raise the suspicion of MEN1. MEN2 should also be considered.

## DIAGNOSIS
### Parathyroid

Hyperparathyroidism is documented by hypercalcemia in the context of an inappropriately high serum PTH. Localization with $Tc^{99m}$ sestamibi can also be helpful although not necessary as all four glands need to be examined intraoperatively, regardless. This test might be more useful in recurrent hyperparathyroidism.

### Entero-pancreatic

Diagnostic testing usually involves showing abnormal levels of the hormone(s) produced. Serum gastrin, fasting glucose, insulin, proinsulin, or chromogranin A can be measured. If suspicious, further specific testing can be done such as a stimulated gastrin (with calcium or secretin) for gastrinoma and 72-hour fast for insulinoma. Ultrasound is frequently used in evaluating pancreatic islet tumors (**217**, **218**), while somatostatin receptor scintigraphy can be used for other neuroendocrine tumors; however, there are few published data describing their use in MEN1.

### Pituitary

Hormonal studies including PRL, IGF-1, and imaging with MRI of the sella (**219**) should be done periodically. If clinically suspicious of an ACTH-producing tumor, screening for hypercortisolism should be performed.

## MANAGEMENT/TREATMENT

Treatment of MEN1 depends on the specific endocrinopathies and severity. Patients with PHP usually require surgery. However, the best timing of surgery is still debated; early parathyroidectomy would minimize the complications of excess PTH, while delaying surgery may promote a simpler operation. Because usually three or all four parathyroid glands are involved, the surgical procedure of choice is a three and a half, subtotal parathyroidectomy, leaving behind a small parathyroid remnant *in situ* or grafted to the

forearm. This is often done with thymectomy because of a higher incidence of a supernumerary parathyroid in the thymus, or thymic carcinoid. Because PHP is estimated to recur in 50% of patients by 12 years, another less favored option would be a total parathyroidectomy and lifelong treatment with vitamin D analogs.

Functional entero-pancreatic tumors are usually sensitive to medications; proton-pump inhibitors or histamine blockers can be used for gastrinomas, while somatostatin analogs can be used for other the other tumors. Surgery is necessary for insulinomas (**220**). Figures **221**, **222** show resected and scan of pancreatic

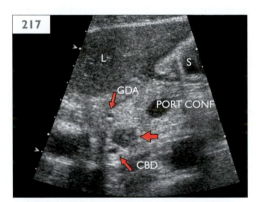

**217** Transabdominal ultrasound showing a hypo-echoic mass in the head of the pancreas (large arrow) classic for an insulinoma. CBD: common bile duct; GDA: gastric duodenal artery; L: liver; Port Conf: confluence of portal veins; S: stomach.

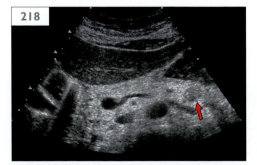

**218** Insulinoma. A 1.4 cm hypoechoic mass (arrow) in the tail of the pancreas.

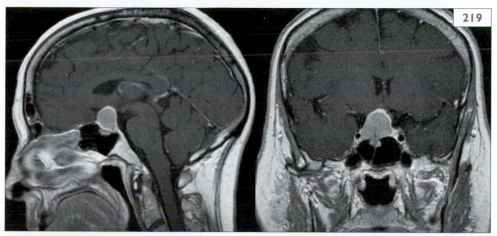

**219** Pituitary macroadenoma measuring 1.5 × 1.9 × 1.8 cm, with slight elevation of the optic chiasm and invasion into the right cavernous sinus seen on MRI.

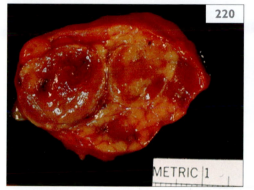

**220** Insulinoma, resected.

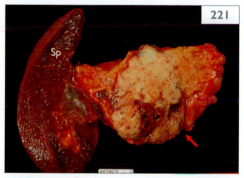

**221** Tail of resected pancreas glucagonoma (arrow) from a patient with MEN1. Spleen (Sp) is seen on the left.

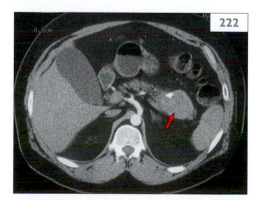

**222** Pancreatic glucagonoma. A 6 cm solid mass with peripheral calcification at the tail of the pancreas is seen.

glucagonoma, respectively. Pancreatic cystic islet cell tumor in a MEN1 patient is shown in **223A–D, 224**. Because of metastatic potential of even small islet tumors (**225**), some centers do recommend early surgery in asymptomatic patients although there is no consensus for this.

The management of pituitary adenomas in MEN1 patients is the same as those with sporadic non-MEN1 pituitary adenomas. It is recommended that kindred of MEN1 patients undergo biochemical evaluation as well as testing for MEN1 germline mutation, although this can be negative in 10–20% of cases. MEN1 carriers should undergo periodic biochemical and radiologic testing. *Table 28* lists the recommended tests for tumor expression in these patients.

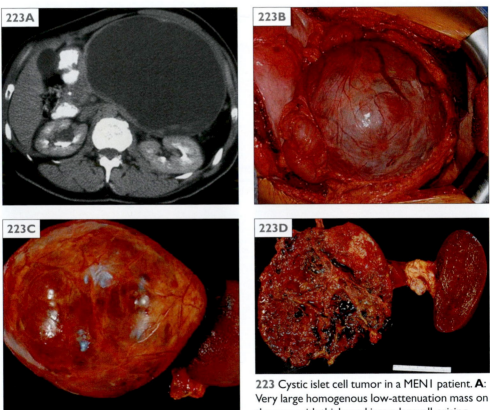

**223** Cystic islet cell tumor in a MEN1 patient. **A**: Very large homogenous low-attenuation mass on the scan with thickened irregular wall, arising from the body of the pancreas; **B**: intraoperative photograph; **C**: gross resected pancreas, with tumor on the left, spleen on the right; **D**: dissected tumor on the left, spleen on the right.

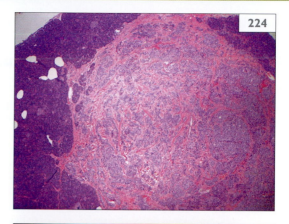

**224** Well-circumscribed pancreatic tumor composed of ribbons and cords of uniform appearing neuroendocrine cells amongst a background of fibrous stroma. The adjacent benign pancreatic parenchyma is present.

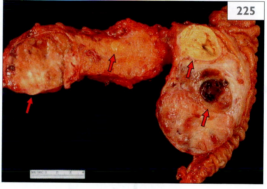

**225** Multiple pancreatic islet cell tumors (arrows).

**Table 28 Recommended tests for tumor expression in a highly likely carrier of MEN1 mutation**

| Tumor | Age to begin (yr) | Biochemical tests annually | Imaging tests every 3 yr |
|---|---|---|---|
| Parathyroid adenoma | 8 | Calcium (especially CA++), PTH | None |
| Gastrinoma | 20 | Gastrin, gastric acid output[a], secretin-stimulated gastrin[a] | None |
| Insulinoma | 5 | Fasting glucose, insulin | |
| Other entero-pancreatic | 20 | Chromogranin-A, glucagon, proinsulin | [111]In-DTP octreotide scan, CT or MRI |
| Anterior pituitary | 5 | PRL, IGF-1 | MRI |
| Foregut carcinoid[b] | 20 | None | CT |

[a]Gastric acid output is measured if gastrin is high; secretin-stimulated gastrin is measured if gastrin is high or if gastric acid output is high.

[b]Stomach is best evaluated for carcinoids (EClomas) incidental to gastric endoscopy. Thymus is removed partially at parathyroidectomy in MEN1. CT: computed tomography; IGF-1: insulin-like growth factor-1; MRI: magnetic resonance imaging; PRL: prolactin; PTH: parathyroid hormone.

(Reprinted from Brandi ML, *et al.* Guidelines for diagnosis and therapy of MEN type I and type 2. *J Clin Endocrinol Metab* 2001;**86**:5658–71. Copyright 2001, The Endocrine Society, with permission.)

# Multiple endocrine neoplasia type 2

## DEFINITION/OVERVIEW

Multiple endocrine neoplasia type 2 (MEN2) represents an autosomal dominant group of disorders classified into three distinct syndromes: MEN2A, MEN2B, and familial medullary thyroid cancer (FMTC). These are rare hereditary cancer syndromes with a high degree of penetrance and variable expression (online Mendelian inheritance in men 171400 and 162300). Their estimated prevalence is 2.5 in 100,000 in the general population.

## PATHOPHYSIOLOGY

MEN2 is due to hereditary germ-line activating point mutations in the *RET* ('rearranged during transfection') proto-oncogene located on chromosome 10 and encoding a plasma membrane-bound tyrosine kinase enzyme. *RET* is expressed in the C-cells of the thyroid, adrenal medulla, and other tissue derived from neural crest. The majority of the mutations in families with FMTC or MEN2A result in the replacement of one of several cysteine residues in the extracellular domain of the molecule. In contrast, all subjects with MEN2B studied so far have had a single mutation in exon 16, in the intracellular catalytic domain of the molecule (**226A**).

Sequencing of DNA for *RET* mutation testing is available and 98% of index MEN2 cases have a *RET* mutation that was identified. Genetic testing has become the preferred screening test for early detection of patients at risk. After a *RET* mutation is found in an index case, all family members with unknown status should be genotyped for the mutation found. Screening family members in MEN2 kindreds is essential because MTC and pheochromocytoma are life-threatening and they can be prevented and cured by early thyroidectomy and adrenalectomy. With improved screening and management of pheochromocytoma, MTC has become the main cause of mortality in MEN2. There is a clear genotype/phenotype correlation in MEN2 groups, such that a specific *RET* codon mutation correlates with the MEN2 syndromic variant, the age of onset of MTC (**226B**), and the aggressiveness of MTC.

## CLINICAL PRESENTATION

MEN2A (Sipple's syndrome) is characterized by predisposition to MTC in over 90%, unilateral or bilateral pheochromocytoma in 50%, and hyperparathyroidism in 20–30% of adult MEN2A gene carriers. Variants of this syndrome are MEN2A with Hirschsprung's disease and MEN2A with cutaneous lichen amyloidosis, presenting as pruritic lesions located on the upper back.

In common with MEN2A, MEN2B has a heritable predisposition to MTC and pheochromocytomas. PHP is not part of this syndrome. MTC is usually more aggressive and develops earlier than in MEN2A and FMTC. Other components of this syndrome are marfanoid body habitus, unusual facies due to coarse features and multiple mucocutaneous ganglioneuromas of tongue, lips, eyelids, and intestine (**227A, B, 228A, B**). Chronic constipation and megacolon are common. Hypertrophy of the corneal nerves can be identified by slit-lamp examination.

FMTC is characterized by a strong predisposition to MTC and the absence of other clinical manifestations of MEN2A or 2B. Many FMTC and MEN2A patients may carry identical *RET* mutations; careful screening needs to be performed in order to differentiate FMTC from MEN2A patients based on medical history and the number of carriers in the kindred, to avoid the risk of overlooking pheochromocytomas.

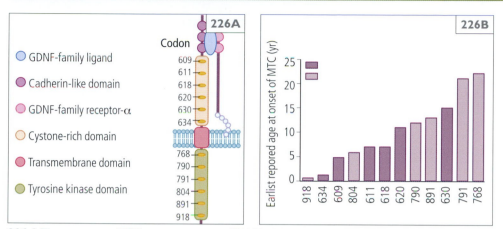

226 **A** The structure of *RET* proto-oncogene. GDNF: glial cell line-derived neurotrophic factor; **B**: the earliest reported age at the onset of medullary thyroid cancer, according to the *RET* mutation. (From Cote GJ, Gagel RF. Lessons learned from the management of a rare genetic cancer. *N Engl J Med* 2003;**349**(16):1566–68. Copyright 2003 Massachusetts Medical Society. All rights reserved.)

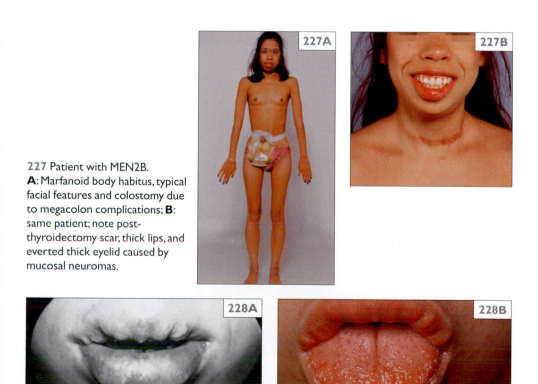

227 Patient with MEN2B. **A**: Marfanoid body habitus, typical facial features and colostomy due to megacolon complications; **B**: same patient; note post-thyroidectomy scar, thick lips, and everted thick eyelid caused by mucosal neuromas.

228 Neuromas in MEN2B. **A**: Thick, lumpy lips; **B**: mucosal neuromas of the tongue and lips.

## MTC in MEN2

### DEFINITION/PATHOPHYSIOLOGY

MTC is a rare neuroendocrine tumor of the parafollicular cells (C-cells) of the thyroid gland. Calcitonin is the primary secretory product of MTC. Multifocal C-cell hyperplasia (CCH) is a precursor lesion to hereditary MTC.

### CLINICAL PRESENTATION

MTC in MEN2 patients is typically multicentric and bilateral (**229**) and presents clinically with a thyroid nodule or cervical adenopathy. The basal serum calcitonin correlates with the tumor mass and is high in patients with palpable tumor. Calcitonin may be normal and may increase only after stimulation tests with calcium or pentagastrin infusion (the latter is no longer available for clinical use in the US) in patients with small tumors or CCH only. Other peptides (ACTH, serotonin, histamine, and others) can be secreted by these tumors; a less common presentation of MTC is related to diarrhea, flushing, or CS due to secretion of some of these peptides.

### DIAGNOSIS

Fine-needle aspiration (FNA) of thyroid nodules or cervical lymph nodes followed by appropriate immunostaining confirms the findings (**230A, B**). Microscopically, MTC appears as nests of neoplastic cells often with amyloid deposits (**231**) and calcifications. The presence of CCH precedes the development of MTC (**232A, B**). Genetic testing for *RET* proto-oncogene has replaced screening with pentagastrin or calcium stimulated calcitonin, allowing earlier and reliable diagnosis. Calcitonin remains an important tumor marker, essential for the follow-up of MTC and also for diagnostic purposes in the small number of families without detectable *RET* mutation. Basal or stimulated calcitonin level is elevated in MTC; the elevated calcitonin after surgery represents the first sign of persistent or recurrent disease.

Staging of MTC is based on TNM system and should be performed preoperatively biochemically, by measurement of calcitonin and CEA, and radiologically with neck ultrasound (**233A, B**) and, if needed, CT scan, MRI neck, chest, and abdomen.

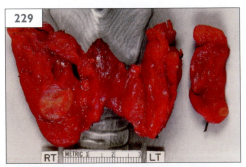

**229** Pathologic specimen from a thyroidectomy. Right MTC (1.5 cm) and multiple small foci of MTC in a patient with MEN2A.

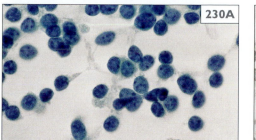

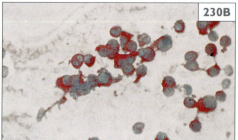

**230** FNA of a thyroid mass in a 65-year-old patient diagnosed with FMTC.  **A**: Spindle-shaped cells, typical for MTC (H&E ×300); **B**: positive calcitonin immunostaining, consistent with MTC (H&E ×150).

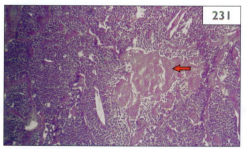

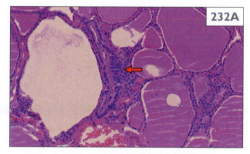

**231** MTC in a patient with MEN2A. Focal amyloid deposits (arrow) (H&E ×100).

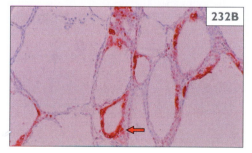

**232** C-cell hyperplasia in a 29-year-old patient with FMTC. **A**: Foci (arrow) (H&E ×20); **B**: foci of C-cell hyperplasia identified by positive calcitonin immunostaining (×20).

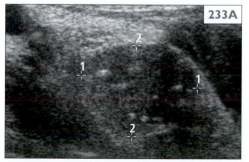

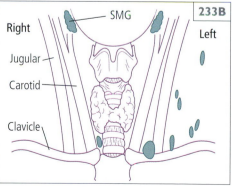

**233** Ultrasound of thyroid. **A**: A 1.9 × 1.5 × 1.2 cm rounded echogenic node is present in the inferior aspect of the left neck just lateral to the left carotid artery, worrisome for metastatic involvement and containing multiple echogenic foci. MTC involvement of this node was proven after FNA; **B**: mapping of suspicious lymph nodes based on the ultrasound of neck in (**A**). SMG: submandibular salivary gland.

Metastatic disease is frequently found when patients present with palpable masses. When metastatic disease is suspected based on CT, more extensive search for the source of disease is performed with additional imaging such as bone scan, octreotide scan, selective venous catheterization, and laparoscopy (**234A, B**).

### MANAGEMENT/TREATMENT
Cure of MTC can be achieved by total thyroidectomy with prophylactic central compartment node dissection and more aggressive neck dissection when metastases to lateral neck lymph nodes are present. If distant metastases are present, palliative surgical intervention with tumor debulking can be considered for management of diarrhea. Chemotherapy and radiation therapy have not been beneficial in the treatment of metastatic MTC. Some patients with metastatic MTC may remain asymptomatic for many years.

### PROGNOSIS
Management of MTC in MEN2 improved dramatically after the discovery of the genes involved. The decision to perform prophylactic thyroidectomy based on *RET* mutation testing alters the clinical course of MTC; early thyroidectomy can be curative in MEN2 and likely increases life expectancy. Prophylactic surgery was recommended based on the youngest age at the first diagnosis of MTC according to specific codon. Patients are grouped in risk categories and recommendations regarding timing of thyroidectomy can be reviewed in recently published consensus guidelines.

## Pheochromocytoma in MEN2

Pheochromocytomas in MEN2A and 2B are often bilateral and usually appear after development of MTC. They are usually benign and intra-adrenal. The penetrance of pheochromocytoma is very variable.

### DIAGNOSIS
Patients at risk are evaluated for clinical symptoms and signs and should undergo annual screening with plasma metanephrines or urinary fractionated catecholamines and metanephrines. Patients who present with MTC or hyperparathyroidism first should be screened for pheochromocytoma prior to surgery and, if found, the pheochromocytoma needs to be addressed first. Imaging of the abdomen with CT (**235**) or MRI for localizations of the tumor is performed and the possibility of bilateral disease should be considered. Radiographic abnormality may present before any clinical or laboratory abnormality (**236**).

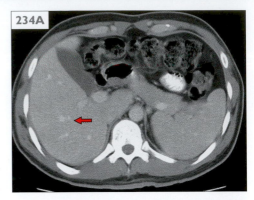

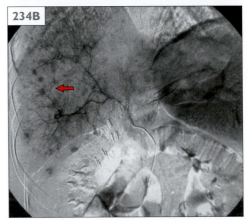

**234** Metastatic MTC. **A**: CT scan of abdomen. Hepatic lesions (arrow) suspicious of metastatic MTC are shown in a patient with MEN2A; **B**: hepatic angiogram identifying metastases of MTC to liver (arrow), confirmed by biopsy.

## MANAGEMENT/TREATMENT

Unilateral or bilateral adrenalectomy (237) is performed usually laparoscopically after pharmacologic preparation. This can be achieved by alpha-adrenergic blockade with phenoxy-benzamine after ensuring the patient is volume-expanded, starting at a dose of 20 mg daily in divided doses, and increasing until goal blood pressure is achieved. Following this, beta-blockade can be initiated. In addition, some groups also utilize metyrosine, a tyrosine hydroxylase inhibitor, to decrease catecholamine production concurrently preoperatively. Following surgery, patients may have up to 50% recurrence rate in the contralateral adrenal. Unilateral adrenalectomy followed by continued surveillance for recurrence in the remaining adrenal is preferred in order to avoid adrenal insufficiency and the need for chronic gluco-corticoid and mineralocorticoid treatment.

## Primary hyperparathyroidism in MEN2A

PHP in MEN2A appears to be milder than in MEN1. Most patients present with asymptomatic hypercalcemia or kidney stones. It is almost always due to multiglandular disease. Periodic screening with serum calcium, annually in families with high prevalence of PHP, is recommended. Management is similar to sporadic hyperparathyroidism except that preoperative localization studies are not needed and all parathyroid glands need to be identified at surgery. Prophylactic subtotal parathyroidec-tomy is not recommended due to the availability of effective treatment and low penetrance of PHP in this syndrome. *RET* testing is not indicated in apparent sporadic hyperparathyroidism in the absence of other clinical suspicion for hereditary MEN2A.

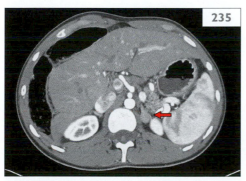

**235** CT scan of abdomen in a patient with MEN2B. The 2 cm left adrenal pheochromocytoma (arrow) was subsequently removed with laparoscopic adrenalectomy.

**236** CT of abdomen. Left adrenal nodule (arrow) in an asymptomatic patient with MEN2A. Biochemistry was negative for pheochromocytoma. Note surgical clips from previous right adrenalectomy due to pheochromocytoma.

**237** Pathologic specimen. A 3.5 cm pheochromocytoma removed by laparoscopic adrenalectomy. Note the very vascular and dusky tumor, typical for pheochromocytoma.

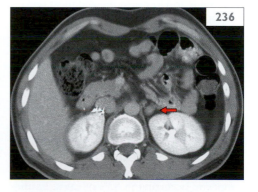

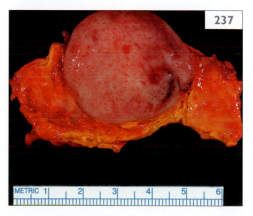

# Carcinoid syndrome

## DEFINITION/OVERVIEW

Carcinoid syndrome describes a constellation of symptoms including flushing, diarrhea, and bronchospasm, arising from tumoral secretion of a variety of biogenic amines and peptides. The incidence for carcinoid tumor is 38.4 per million, although carcinoid syndrome is seen in only about 10% of patients with carcinoid tumors. Most carcinoid tumors are found in the gastrointestinal tract (54.5%) with the small bowel being the most common location, followed by the pulmonary tree (30.1%).

## ETIOLOGY

Symptoms are caused by the secretion of biogenic amines and peptides such as serotonin, 5-hydroxytryptophan, kallikrien, histamine, prostaglandins, and VIP. Over 40 types of secretory products have been implicated in carcinoid tumors.

## PATHOPHYSIOLOGY

Carcinoids are slow growing and most remain asymptomatic. Symptoms are related to the dominant culprit substance. Secretion of serotonin or its precursors cause bowel hypermotility and secretory diarrhea. This also causes fibrosis which is thought to be the mechanism of carcinoid valvular disease. Histamine, kallikrein, and prostaglandin secretion cause peripheral vasodilation leading to spells of flushing and even hypotension.

## CLINICAL PRESENTATION

Secretory diarrhea is the most common symptom, occurring in 83% of cases. Fasting does not ameliorate the diarrhea. A dry cutaneous flushing is seen in about half of patients presenting with carcinoid syndrome. This may occur spontaneously or as a result of alcohol or tyramine-containing foods, and typically lasts seconds to minutes. Midgut carcinoids usually cause the classic upper body flushing of a pink to red hue, while foregut carcinoids may cause a more intense violaceous flush with telangiectasia. Over time, facial skin thickening with a leonine appearance may be observed in these patients. The vasodilatory effect may be so pronounced that it leads to systemic hypotension, dizziness, and tachycardia.

Other symptoms include dyspnea, wheezing, or bronchospasm in 20% of patients. Carcinoid valvular disease is rare but may be seen in up to 60% of patients with metastatic carcinoid. The right heart is usually involved with tricuspid and pulmonary valve damage (**238A, B**). Other less common symptoms occurring in association with carcinoid tumors include CS (from an ACTH-producing carcinoid), muscle wasting, and peptic ulcer disease although these are not considered to be part of carcinoid syndrome *per se*. Liver metastasis is shown in figures **239, 240** and bronchial carcinoid in **241**.

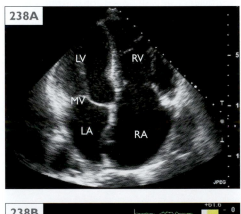

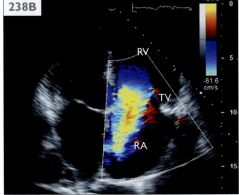

**238** Carcinoid valvuvar disease. **A**: Tricuspid regurgitation. The tricuspid valve (TV) is thickened and open during ventricular systole, in comparison to closed mitral valve (MV); **B**: severe tricuspid regurgitation as seen on color doppler (regurgitant jet in blue).

## DIFFERENTIAL DIAGNOSIS

Menopause, or medications simulating menopause such as GnRH analogs or antiestrogens, alcohol consumption especially with disulfiram, pheochromocytoma, MTC, systemic mastocytosis, polycythemia rubra vera.

## DIAGNOSIS

Elevated 24-hour urinary 5-hydroxy-indoleacetic acid (5-HIAA) results from the breakdown of serotonin. Foregut carcinoids may produce less serotonin and therefore the urine may contain relatively little 5-HIAA; 5-hydroxytryptophan (5-HTP) may be elevated instead. Chromogranin A can be checked as well, although this is not specific for carcinoid tumors.

Octreotide scan appears to have the greatest sensitivity, followed by CT and MRI. Transthoracic or transesophageal echocardiogram can be used to aid diagnosis and determining the prognosis of patients with carcinoid valvular disease.

## MANAGEMENT/TREATMENT

Octreotide, a somatostatin analog, is used for symptomatic treatment of carcinoid syndrome. Other agents such as corticosteroids, phenoxybenzamine, and cyproheptadine have been used with less success. Antidiarrheals or opioids can also improve diarrhea, while bronchospasm may respond to albuterol.

Avoidance of triggers such as alcohol and certain foods should be emphasized. Because carcinoid is indolent, most patients have metastatic disease when they present with the syndrome. Surgery or hepatic artery embolization can be carried out to palliate severe symptoms.

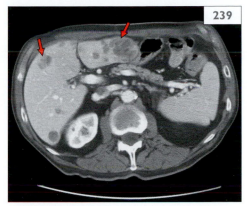

**239** Multiple low-attenuation masses in both lobes of the liver in a patient with metastatic carcinoid tumor. Carcinoids typically are vascular in the arterial phase and have higher-attenuation.

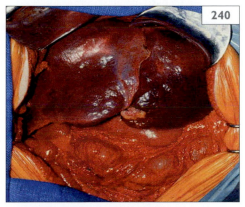

**240** Carcinoid metastasis to liver.

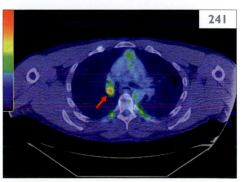

**241** Bronchial carcinoid, manifesting as a 1.6 cm mass adjacent to the right bronchus (arrow) with moderate FDG uptake on PET.

# Autoimmune polyglandular syndromes

## DEFINITION/ETIOLOGY

Autoimmune polyglandular syndrome (APS) is a hereditary, diverse group of clinical syndromes of endocrine deficiencies caused by autoantibody-mediated destruction of endocrine and nonendocrine organs.

APS type I, also called autoimmune polyendocrinopathy, candidiasis, ectodermal dystrophy (APECED) syndrome, is inherited in an autosomal recessive fashion and is associated with a mutation in the autoimmune regulator gene (AIRE) on chromosome 21q22.3. This usually presents in early childhood.

APS type II, also called Schmidt's syndrome, is likely polygenic and is more prevalent than APS type I. There is a female predominance and the disease tends to manifest during adulthood.

## PATHOPHYSIOLOGY

Autoantibodies to various components of affected organs have been implicated. These include antibodies to adrenocortical enzymes such as 21-hydroxylase or 17-alpha-hydroxylase, glutamic acid decarboxylase (GAD), islet cell antibodies (ICA), TPO, and thyroglobulin. This leads to inhibition of enzymatic activities or immune destruction of the gland and endocrine insufficiency. In addition, patients often have reduced systemic cell-mediated immunity. Infections are common in APS type I.

## CLINICAL PRESENTATION

Characterizing APS can be challenging due to the large heterogeneity and overlap of clinical manifestations and the broad spectrum.

### APS type I

Hypoparathyroidism and chronic mucocutaneous candidiasis are seen in up to 80% of patients with APS type I and are usually the first manifestations, occurring in early childhood. Primary adrenal insufficiency is the next most common, seen in 67%. Other manifestations include primary hypogonadism, type 1 diabetes mellitus, autoimmune gastritis and other gastrointestinal problems, skin conditions such as alopecia and vitiligo, keratoconjunctivitis, autoimmune hepatitis, and thyroid disease (less common than in APS type II). Ectodermal dystrophies may manifest as tooth enamel hypoplasia and nail dystrophy.

### APS type II

Unlike APS type I, APS type II usually manifests in adulthood, most commonly in the third and fourth decades of life and is at least three times more common in females. Almost all patients develop adrenal insufficiency, while autoimmune thyroid disease is seen in up to 70% of APS type II and type 1 diabetes mellitus in half. Autoimmune adrenal insufficiency or Addison's disease is usually the initial presenting feature, although many are found to have concomitant type 1 diabetes mellitus and/or autoimmune thyroid disease at presentation. Other less common features include pernicious anemia, primary gonadal failure, and skin disease.

Table 29 lists the differences between APS types I and II. Some groups classify the above autoimmune endocrinopathies in the absence of adrenal insufficiency as APS type III, although others consider that to be early type II before Addison's disease sets in.

## DIFFERENTIAL DIAGNOSIS

Autoimmune and nonimmune endocrinopathies also occur together in other conditions such as POEMS (polyneuropathy, organomegaly, endocrinopathy, M protein, skin changes) syndrome, Wolfram's syndrome, Kearns–Sayre syndrome, chromosomal abnormalities (trisomy 21, Turner's syndrome), and thymomas.

## DIAGNOSIS

There is no universally accepted diagnostic protocol for APS. However, once APS is suspected, testing for autoantibodies is indicated. Organ-specific autoantibodies predict for pre-existing, or a potential for, insufficiency of that endocrine gland. These include ICA and GAD for type 1 diabetes, TPO for thyroid disease, 21-hydroxylase for Addison's disease, and anti-smooth muscle antibody for autoimmune hepatitis.

Endocrine organ-specific function can be evaluated by measuring fasting glucose (pancreas), calcium and phosphorus (PTH if indicated), TSH, early morning cortisol, gonadotropins with sex steroids, and hemoglobin (pernicious anemia). In the presence of autoantibodies, endocrine organ function should be evaluated at least annually.

## MANAGEMENT/TREATMENT

Treatment of the hormonal deficiencies in APS is similar to that of the sporadic types. However, the physician must be astute to the possibility of multiorgan involvement, as treatment of hypothyroidism preceding corticosteroid replacement in undiagnosed adrenal insufficiency may precipitate an Addisonian crisis. Also, inexplicable decreasing insulin requirements in a patient with type 1 diabetes may hint at developing adrenal insufficiency or hypothyroidism.

Mucocutaneous candidiasis is treated by antifungal lozenges or, in severe cases, systemic antifungals such as fluconazole or ketoconazole. Good oral hygiene and avoidance of orthodontic devices are important. Chronic mucocutaneous candidiasis increases the risk of oral cancer. Immunosuppressants, such as prednisone, azathioprine, and cyclosporine, are used for the treatment of autoimmune hepatitis.

**Table 29 Comparison of APS types I and II**

| | APS I (%) | APS II (%) |
|---|---|---|
| Comparative frequency | Less common | More common |
| Onset | Infancy/early childhood | Late childhood/adulthood |
| Heredity | Autosomal recessive | Polygenic |
| Gender | Males = females | Female predominance |
| Genetics | AIRE gene; no HLA association | HLA associated; DR/DQ |
| Hypoparathyroidism | 77–89 | None |
| Mucocutaneous candidiasis | 73–100 | None |
| Ectodermal dysplasia | 77 | None |
| Addison's disease | 60–86 | 70–100 |
| Type 1 diabetes | 4–18 | 41–52 |
| Autoimmune thyroid disease | 8–10 | 70 |
| Pernicious anemia | 12–15 | 2–25 |
| Gonadal failure | | |
| • Females | 30–60 | 3.5–10 |
| • Males | 7–17 | 5 |
| Vitiligo | 4–13 | 4–5 |
| Alopecia | 27 | 2 |
| Autoimmune hepatitis | 10–15 | Rare |
| Malabsorption | 10–18 | Rare |

(Reprinted from *Endocrinol Metab Clin N Am* 2002;**31**. Schatz DA, Winter WE. Autoimmune polyglandular syndrome II: clinical syndrome and treatment, pp. 339–52. Copyright 2002, with permission from Elsevier.)

## Chapter 1

Castro MR, Gharib H. Continuing controversies in the management of thyroid nodules. *Ann Intern Med* 2005;**142**(11):926–31.

Cooper DS (ed). Medical Management of Thyroid Disease. Marcel Dekker, New York, 2001.

Cooper DS, Doherty GM, Haugen BR, *et al.* Management guidelines for patients with thyroid nodules and differentiated thyroid cancer. *Thyroid* 2006;**16**(2):109–42.

DeGroot LJ (ed). *The Thyroid and Its Diseases*. (www.thyroidmanager.org/thyroidbook. htm): 2008. Endocrine Education Inc., South Dartmouth.

Mandel SJ. Diagnostic use of ultrasonography in patients with nodular thyroid disease. *Endocr Pract* 2004;**10**(3):246–52.

Weetman AP. Graves' disease. *N Engl J Med* 2000;**343**(17):1236–48.

## Chapter 2

American Diabetes Association position statement. Preventive foot care in diabetes. *Diabetes Care* 2004;**27**(Supplement 1):S63–4.

Boulton AJ, Vinik AI, Arezzo JC, *et al.* Diabetic neuropathies: a statement by the American Diabetes Association. *Diabetes Care* 2005;**28**:956–62.

Burke JP, Hale DE, Hazuda HP, Stern MP. A quantitative scale of acanthosis nigricans. *Diabetes Care* 1999;**22**:1655–9.

Fong DS, Aiello LP, Ferris FL, Klein R. Diabetic retinopathy. *Diabetes Care* 2004;**27**:2540–53.

Freeman R. Autonomic peripheral neuropathy. *Lancet* 2005;**365**:1259–70.

Gross JL, deAzevedo MJ, Silveiro SP, Canani LH, Caramori ML, Zelmanovitz T. Diabetic nephropathy: diagnosis, prevention, and treatment. *Diabetes Care* 2005;**28**:164–76.

Mayfield JA, Reiber GE, Sanders LJ, Janisse, D, Pogach M. Preventive foot care in people with diabetes. *Diabetes Care* 1998;**21**:2161–77.

Shepherd J, Barter P, Carmena R, *et al.* Effect of lowering LDL cholesterol substantially below currently recommended levels in patients with coronary heart disease and diabetes: the Treating to New Targets (TNT) Study. *Diabetes Care* 2006;**29**:1220–6.

Vinik AI, Maser RE, Mitchell BD, Freeman R. Diabetic autonomic neuropathy. *Diabetes Care* 2003;**26**:1553–79.

Waters DD, Guyton JR, Herrington DM, McGowan MP, Wenger NK, Shear C. TNT Steering Committee members and investigators. Treating to New Targets (TNT) Study: does lowering low-density lipoprotein cholesterol levels below currently recommended guidelines yield incremental clinical benefit? *Am J Cardiol* 2004;**93**:154–8.

## Chapter 3

AACE/AAES Task Force on primary hyperparathyroidism. The American Association of Clinical Endocrinologists and the American Association of Endocrine Surgeons position statement on the diagnosis and management of primary hyperparathyroidism. *Endocr Prac* 2005;**11**(1):49-54.

Balemans W, Van Wesenbeeck L, Van Hul W. A clinical and molecular overview of the human osteopetroses. *Calcified Tissue Int* 2005;77:263–74.

Bastepe M, Jüppner H. GNAS locus and pseudohypoparathyroidism. *Hormone Res* 2005;63:65–74.

Dawson-Hughes B, Gold DT, Rodbard HW, Bonner FJ Jr, Khosla S, Swift SS. *Physician's Guide to the Prevention and Treatment of Osteoporosis*. National Osteoporosis Foundation, 2003. www.nof.org/physguide/index.htm.

Leib ES, Lewiecki EM, Binkley N, Hamdy RC, International Society for Clinical Densitometry. Official positions of the International Society for Clinical Densitometry. *J Clin Densit* 2004;7:1–6.

Lyles KW, Siris ES, Singer FR, Meunier PJ. A clinical approach to the diagnosis and management of Paget's disease of bone. *J Bone Min Res* 2001;16:1379–87.

Marx SJ. Hyperparathyroid and hypoparathyroid disorders. *N Engl J Med* 2000;343(25):1863–75.

Mauck KF, Clarke BL. Diagnosis, screening, prevention, and treatment of osteoporosis. *Mayo Clin Proc* 2006;81(5):662–72.

Nelson HD, Helfand M, Woolf SH, Allan JD. Screening for postmenopausal osteoporosis: a review of the evidence for the US Preventive Services Task Force. *Ann Intern Med* 2002;137:529–41.

NIH Consensus Development Panel on osteoporosis prevention, diagnosis and therapy. Osteoporosis prevention, diagnosis, and therapy. *JAMA* 2001;285:785–95.

Ott S. Osteoporosis and bone physiology. 2006, http://courses.washington.edu/bonephys/ophome.html

Roodman GD. Mechanisms of bone metastasis. *N Engl J Med* 2004;350(16):1655–64.

Roodman GD, Windle JJ. Paget disease of the bone. *J Clin Investig* 2005;115(2):200–8.

Sambook P, Cooper C. Osteoporosis. *Lancet* 2006;367:2010–18.

Silverberg SJ, Shane E, Jacobs TP, Siris E, Bilezikian JP. A 10-year prospective study of primary hyperparathyroidism with or without parathyroid surgery. *N Engl J Med* 1999;341(17):1249–55.

Tolar J, Teitelbaum SL, Orchard PJ. Osteopetrosis. *N Engl J Med* 2004;351(27):2839–49.

White MP. Paget's disease of the bone. *N Engl J Med* 2006;355(6):593–600.

WHO Scientific Group on the prevention and management of osteoporosis. *Prevention and Management of Osteoporosis: Report of a WHO Scientific Group*. Publications of the World Health Organization, Geneva, 2003.

# Chapter 4

Bichet DG. Diabetes insipidus and vasopressin. In: Moore WT, Eastman RC (eds). *Diagnostic Endocrinology*. BC Decker, Toronto, 1990, pp. 111–24.

Biermasz NR, van Dulken H, Roelfsema F. Ten-year follow-up results of trans-sphenoidal microsurgery in acromegaly. *J Clin Endocrinol Metab* 2000;85:4596–602.

Chandrasekharappa SC, Teh BT. Functional studies of the MEN1 gene. *J Intern Med* 2003;253(6):606–15.

Katznelson L, Klibanski A. Prolactin and its disorders. In: *Principles and Practice of Endocrinology and Metabolism*, 2nd edn. JB Lippincott, Philadelphia, 1995.

Kreutzer J, Vance ML, Lopes MB, Laws ER Jr. Surgical management of GH-secreting pituitary adenomas: an outcome study using modern remission criteria. *J Clin Endocrinol Metab* 2001;86:4072–7.

Krupp P, Monka C. Bromocriptine during pregnancy: safety aspects. *Klin Wochenschr* 1987;**65**:823–7.

Marx SJ, Simonds W. Hereditary hormone excess: genes, molecular pathways, and syndromes. *Endocr Rev* 2003: **26**(5):615–61.

Melmed S. Acromegaly. *N Engl J Med* 1990;**322**:966–77.

Molitch ME, Thorner MO, Wilson C. Therapeutic controversy: management of prolactinomas. *J Clin Endocrinol Metab* 1997;**82**:996.

Molitch ME, Clemmons DR, Malozowski S, *et al*. for The Endocrine Society's Clinical Guidelines Subcommittee. Evaluation and treatment of adult growth hormone deficiency: an Endocrine Society clinical practice guideline. *J Clin Endocrinol Metab* 2006;**91**:1621–34.

Sam S, Molitch ME. The pituitary mass: diagnosis and management. *Rev Endocr Metab Disor* 2005;**6**(1):55–62.

Thorner MO, Vance ML, Kaws ER, *et al*. The anterior pituitary. In: Wilson JD, Foster DW (eds). *Williams Text Book of Endocrinology*, 9th edn. WB Saunders, Philadelphia, 1998, pp. 249–340.

Vance ML. Hypopituitarism. *N Engl J Med* 1994;**330**:1651–62.

Verbalis JG. Disorders of water metabolism. www.sciencedirect.com/science/journal/ 1521690X *Best Prac Res Clin Endocrinol Metab* 2003;**17**(4):471–503.

Yanovski JA, Cutler GB, Chrousos GP, *et al*. Corticotropin-releasing hormone stimulation following low-dose dexamethasone administration. A new test to distinguish Cushing's syndrome from psuedo-Cushing's states. *JAMA* 1993;**269**:2232–38.

## Chapter 5

Allolio B, Fassnacht M. Clinical review: adrenocortical carcinoma: clinical update. *J Clin Endocrinol Metab* 2006;**91**(6):2027–37.

Bravo EL, Tagle R. Phaeochromocytoma: state-of-the-art and future prospects. *Endocr Rev* 2003;**24**(4):539–53.

Dackiw AP, Lee JE, Gagel RF, Evans DB. Adrenal cortical carcinoma. *World J Surg* 2001;**25**:914–26.

Ganguly A. Primary aldosteronism. *N Engl J Med* 1998;**339**(25):1828-34.

Gopan T, Remer EM, Hamrahian AH. Evaluating and managing adrenal incidentalomas. *Cleveland Clin J Med* 2006;**73**(6):561–8.

Grinspoon SK, Biller BM. Clinical review 62: laboratory assessment of adrenal insufficiency. *J Clin Endocrinol Metab* 1994;**79**(4):923–31.

Grumbach MM, Biller BM, Braunstein GD, *et al*. Management of the clinically inapparent adrenal mass ('incidentaloma'). *Ann Intern Med* 2003;**138**:424–29.

Hamrahian AH, Oseni TS, Arafah BM. Measurements of serum free cortisol in critically ill patients. *N Engl J Med* 2004;**350**(16):1629–38.

Hamrahian AH, Ioachimescu AG, Remer EM, *et al*. Clinical utility of noncontrast computed tomography attenuation value (Hounsfield units) to differentiate adrenal adenomas/hyperplasias from nonadenomas: Cleveland Clinic experience. *J Clin Endocrinol Metab* 2005;**90**(2):871–7.

Ilias I, Pacak K. Current approaches and recommended algorithm for the diagnostic localization of phaeochromocytoma. *J Clin Endocrinol Metab* 2004;**89**(2):479–91.

Kloos RT, Gross MD, Francis IR, Korobkin M, Shapiro B. Incidentally discovered adrenal masses. *Endocr Rev* 1995;**16**:460–84.

Lacroix A, Bourdeau I. Bilateral adrenal Cushing's syndrome: macronodular adrenal hyperplasia and primary pigmented nodular adrenocortical disease. *Endocrinol Metabol Clin N Am* 2005;**34**(2):441–58.

Lenders JW, Pacak K, Walther MM, *et al*. Biochemical diagnosis of phaeochromocytoma: which test is best? *JAMA* 2002;**287**:1427–34.

Lenders JW, Eisenhofer G, Mannelli M, Pacak K. Phaeochromocytoma. *Lancet* 2005;**366**(9486):665–75.

McMahon GT, Dluhy RG. Glucocorticoid-remediable aldosteronism. *Cardiol Rev* 2004;**12**(1):44–8.

Merke DP, Bornstein SR. Congenital adrenal hyperplasia. *Lancet* 2005;**365**:2125– 36.

Oelkers W. Adrenal insufficiency. *N Engl J Med* 1996;**335**(16):1206–12.

White PC, Speiser PW. Congenital adrenal hyperplasia due to 21-hydroxylase deficiency. *Endocr Rev* 2000;**21**:245–91.

Speiser PW, White PC. Congenital adrenal hyperplasia. *N Engl J Med* 2003;**349**:776–88.

Young WF, Jr. Minireview: primary aldosteronism – changing concepts in diagnosis and treatment. *Endocrinology* 2003;**144**(6):2208–13.

## Chapter 6

Azziz R, Carmina E, Dewailly D, *et al*. Criteria for defining polycystic ovary syndrome as a predominantly hyperandrogenic syndrome: an androgen excess society guideline. *J Clin Endocrinol Metab* 2006;**91**(11):4237–45. Epub 2006 Aug 29.

Beck-Peccoz P, Persani L. Premature ovarian failure. *Orphanet J Rare Dis* 2006;**1**:9.

Broekmans FJ, Knauff EA, Valkenburg O, Laven JS, Eijkemans MJ, Fauser BC. PCOS according to the Rotterdam consensus criteria: change in prevalence among WHO-II anovulation and association with metabolic factors. *Br J Obstet Gynaecol* 2006;**113**(10):1210–17.

Bussani C, Papi L, Sestini R, *et al*. Premature ovarian failure and fragile X premutation: a study on 45 women. *Eur J Obstet Gynecol Reprod Biol* 2004;**112**(2):189–91.

Cobin RH, Futterweit W, Nestler JE, *et al*. American Association of Clinical Endocrinologists position statement on metabolic and cardiovascular consequences of polycystic ovary syndrome. *Endocr Practice* 2005;**11**(2):125–34.

Cobin RH and Task Force, American Association of Clinical Endocrinologists. Guidelines for clinical practice for the diagnosis and treatment of menopause. *Endocr Practice* 2006;**12**(3):May/June.

Conte FA, Grumbach MA. Abnormalities of sexual determination and differentiation. In: Greenspan FS and Strewler GJ (eds). *Basic and Clinical Endocrinology*, 5th edn. Appleton and Lange, Stamford, 1997, pp. 487–520.

Delemarre-van de Waal HA. Application of gonadotropin releasing hormone in hypogonadotropic hypogonadism: diagnostic and therapeutic aspects. *Eur J Endocrinol* 2004;**151**(Suppl 3):U89–94.

Essah PA, Apridonidze T, Iuorno MJ, Nestler JE. Effects of short-term and long-term metformin treatment on menstrual cyclicity in women with polycystic ovary syndrome. *Fertil Steril* 2006;**86**(1):230–2. Epub 2006 May 23.

Gordon PR, Kerwin JP, Boesen KG, Senf J. Sertraline to treat hot flashes: a randomized controlled, double-blind, crossover trial in a general population. *Menopause* 2006;**13**(4):568–75.

Guzick DS, Overstreet JW, Factor-Litvak P, *et al*. Sperm morphology, motility and concentration in fertile and infertile men. *N Engl J Med* 2001;**345**:1388–93.

Hodgson SF, Watts NB, Bilezikian JP, *et al*. AACE Osteoporosis Task Force. American Association of Clinical Endocrinologists medical guidelines for clinical practice for the prevention and treatment of postmenopausal osteoporosis: 2001 edition, with selected updates for 2003. *Endocr Practice* 2003;**9**(6):544–64.

Madgar I, Weissenberg R, Lunenfeld B, Karasik A, Goldwasser B. A controlled trial of high spermatic vein ligation for varicocele in infertile men. *Fertil Steril* 1995;**63**:120–4.

Manson JE, Hsia J, Johnson KC, *et al*. Estrogen plus progestin and the risk of coronary heart disease. *N Engl J Med* 2003;**349**(6):523–34.

McCartney CR, Eagleson CA, Marshall JC. Regulation of gonadotropin secretion: implications for polycystic ovary syndrome. *Semin Reprod Med* 2002;**20**(4):317–26.

Neveu N, Granger L, St-Michel P, Lavoie HB. Comparison of clomiphene citrate, metformin, or the combination of both for first-line ovulation induction and achievement of pregnancy in 154 women with polycystic ovary syndrome. *Fertil Steril* 2007;**87**:113–20. Epub 2006 Nov 1.

Pasquali R, Gambineri A. Insulin-sensitizing agents in women with polycystic ovary syndrome. *Fertil Steril* 2006;**86**(Suppl 1):S28–9.

Petak S, Cobin RH. *Reproductive Disorders in Evidence Based Endocrinology*. Mary Ann Liebert, Philadelphia, 2006, pp.125–152.

Rossetti F, Rizzolio F, Pramparo T, *et al*. A susceptibility gene for premature ovarian failure (POF) maps to proximal Xq28. *Eur J Hum Genet* 2004;**12**(10):829–34.

Smith SR, Piacquadio DJ, Beger B, Littler C. Eflornithine cream combined with laser therapy in the management of unwanted facial hair growth in women: a randomized trial. *Dermatol Surg* 2006;**32**(10):1237–43.

Stewart DR, Dombroski BA, Urbanek M, *et al*. Fine mapping of genetic susceptibility to polycystic ovary syndrome on chromosome 19p13.2 and tests for regulatory activity. *J Clin Endocrinol Metab* 2006;**91**(10):4112–7. Epub 2006 Jul 25.

Tsai PS, Gill JC. Mechanisms of disease: insights into X-linked and autosomal-dominant Kallmann syndrome. *Nat Clin Pract Endocrinol Metab* 2006;**2**(3):160–71.

Van Rumste MME, Evers JLH, Fraquhar CM, *et al*. Intra-cytoplasmic sperm injection versus partial zona dissection, subzonal insemination, and conventional techniques for oocyte insemination during in vitro fertilization (Cochrane Review). In: *The Cochrane Library*, Issue 3, 2002. Update Software, Oxford.

Vrbikova J, Hill M, Starka L, *et al*. The effects of long-term metformin treatment on adrenal and ovarian steroidogenesis in women with polycystic ovary syndrome. *Eur J Endocrinol* 2001;**144**(6):619–28.

Witchel SF. Puberty and polycystic ovary syndrome. *Mol Cell Endocrinol* 2006;**25**:254–5; 146–53. Epub 2006 Jun 5. Review.

## Chapter 7

The Long-Term Intervention with Pravastatin in Ischaemic Disease (LIPID) Study Group. Prevention of cardiovascular events and death with pravastatin in patients with coronary heart disease and a broad range of initial cholesterol levels. *N Engl J Med* 1998;**339**:1349–57.

The Scandinavian Simvastatin Survival Study. Randomised trial of cholesterol lowering in 4444 patients with coronary heart disease (4S). *Lancet* 1994;**344**:1383–89.

Ashen MD, Blumenthal RS. Clinical practice. Low HDL cholesterol levels. *N Engl J Med* 2005;**353**:1252–60.

Baigent C, Keech A, Kearney PM, *et al*. Efficacy and safety of cholesterol-lowering treatment: prospective meta-analysis of data from 90,056 participants in 14 randomised trials of statins. *Lancet* 2005;**366**:1267–78.

Downs JR, Clearfield M, Weis S, *et al*. Primary prevention of acute coronary events with lovastatin in men and women with average cholesterol levels: results of AFCAPS/TexCAPS. Air Force/Texas Coronary Atherosclerosis Prevention Study. *JAMA* 1998;**279**:1615–22.

Executive Summary of the Third Report of the National Cholesterol Education Program (NCEP) Expert Panel on detection, evaluation, and treatment of high blood cholesterol in adults (Adult Treatment Panel III). *JAMA* 2001;**285**:2486–97.

Grundy SM, Cleeman JI, Merz CN, *et al*. Implications of recent clinical trials for the National Cholesterol Education Program Adult Treatment Panel III guidelines. *Circulation* 2004;**110**:227–39.

Levine GN, Keaney JF, Jr, Vita JA. Cholesterol reduction in cardiovascular disease. Clinical benefits and possible mechanisms. *N Engl J Med* 1995;**332**:512–21.

MRC/BHF Heart Protection Study of cholesterol lowering with simvastatin in 20,536 high-risk individuals: a randomised placebo-controlled trial. *Lancet* 2002;**360**:7–22.

Nissen SE, Tuzcu EM, Schoenhagen P, *et al*. Effect of intensive compared with moderate lipid-lowering therapy on progression of coronary atherosclerosis: a randomized controlled trial (REVERSAL). *JAMA* 2004;**291**:1071–80.

Rubins HB, Robins SJ, Collins D, *et al*. Gemfibrozil for the secondary prevention of coronary heart disease in men with low levels of high-density lipoprotein cholesterol. Veterans Affairs High-Density Lipoprotein Cholesterol Intervention Trial Study Group. *N Engl J Med* 1999;**341**:410–18.

Sacks FM, Pfeffer MA, Moye LA, *et al*. The effect of pravastatin on coronary events after myocardial infarction in patients with average cholesterol levels. Cholesterol and Recurrent Events Trial Investigators. *N Engl J Med* 1996;**335**:1001–9.

Sever PS, Dahlof B, Poulter NR, *et al*. Prevention of coronary and stroke events with atorvastatin in hypertensive patients who have average or lower-than-average cholesterol concentrations, in the Anglo-Scandinavian Cardiac Outcomes Trial: Lipid Lowering Arm (ASCOT-LLA): a multicentre randomised controlled trial. *Lancet* 2003;**361**:1149–58.

# Chapter 8

Brandi ML, Gagel RF, Angeli A, *et al*. Guidelines for diagnosis and therapy of MEN type 1 and type 2. *J Clin Endocrinol Metab* 2001;**86**(12):5658–71.

Donis-Keller H, Dou S, Chi D, *et al*. Mutations in the RET proto-oncogene are associated with MEN 2A and FMTC. *Hum Mol Genet* 1993;**2**(7):851–6.

Eng C, Clayton D, Schuffenecker I, *et al*. The relationship between specific RET proto-oncogene mutations and disease phenotype in multiple endocrine neoplasia type 2. International RET mutation consortium analysis. *JAMA* 1993;**276**(19):1575–9.

Heshmati HM, Gharib H, van Heerden JA, *et al*. Advances and controversies in the diagnosis and management of medullary thyroid carcinoma. *Am J Med* 1991;**103**(1):60–9.

Kloos RT, Eng C, Evans DE, *et al*. Medullary thyroid cancer: Management Guidelines of the American Thyroid Association. *Thyroid* 2009;**19**:565–612.

Maton P. The carcinoid syndrome. *JAMA* 1988;**260**(11):1602–5.

Modlin IM, Kidd M, Latich I, *et al*. Current status of gastrointestinal carcinoids. *Gastroenterology* 2005;**128**(6):1717–51.

Mulligan LM, Kwok JB, Healey CS, *et al*. Germ-line mutations of the RET proto-oncogene in multiple endocrine neoplasia type 2A. *Nature* 1993;**363**(6428):458–60.

Perheentupa J. APS-I/APECED: the clinical disease and therapy. *Endocrinol Metab Clin N Am* 2002;**31**(2):295–320.

Rizzoli R, Green J, 3rd, Marx SJ. Primary hyperparathyroidism in familial multiple endocrine neoplasia type I. Long-term follow-up of serum calcium levels after parathyroidectomy. *Am J Med* 1985;**78**(3):467–74.

Schatz DA, Winter WE. Autoimmune polyglandular syndrome II: clinical syndrome and treatment. *Endocrinol Metab Clin N Am* 2002;**31**:339–52.

Verges B, Boureille F, Goudet P, *et al*. Pituitary disease in MEN type 1 (MEN1): data from the France-Belgium MEN1 multicenter study. *J Clin Endocrinol Metab* 2002;**87**(2):457–65.

Note: Page numbers in *italic* refer to tables

abdominal aortic aneurysm 179
abetalipoproteinemia (autosomal recessive)
  *176–7*
acanthosis nigricans 49, 103, 150, 151
ACE inhibitors, *see* angiotensin-converting
  enzyme (ACE) inhibitors
acne 138, 151
acromegaly 99–103
  diabetes mellitus 60–1
acropachy, thyroid 16, 18
Addison's disease 115, 204
ADH, *see* antidiuretic hormone
adrenal crisis 119
adrenal glands
  anatomy and physiology 114
  androgen production 136, 137–9, 140
  benign adenomas 62, 120–3, 130
  bilateral macronodular hyperplasia 130,
    131
  lesions in MEN1 191
  steroid biosynthesis 136
adrenal incidentaloma 134, 143–7
adrenal insufficiency 115–19
  after adrenal resection 146
  causes 115, *115*
  critically ill patient 119
  diagnosis 117–19
  differentiation of primary and secondary
    118
  management 119–20
  primary 115, *115*, 204
  secondary 115
adrenal venous sampling 123
adrenalectomy
  Cushing syndrome 135
  laparoscopic 123, 135, 146
  open 142–3
  pheochromocytoma 201
adrenocortical carcinomas (ACCs) 62, 130,
  140–3

adrenocorticotrophic hormone (ACTH)
  92, *93*
  ectopic syndrome 104–6
  serum levels 134
adrenocorticotrophic hormone (ACTH)
  stimulation test 118, 139
adrenoleukodystrophy, X-linked 119
adrenomyeloneuropathy 119
advanced glycosylation end-products 41,
  43, 45
Albright's hereditary osteodystrophy
  (AHO) 75–6, *77*
aldosterone 114
  biosynthesis 114, 136
  hypersecretion 120, 146
  plasma (PAC) 122
  urinary excretion 122, 146
aldosterone-producing adenoma (APA)
  120, 122–3
aldosteronism
  primary 120–3, 146
  secondary 120
alkaline phosphatase levels 79, 82, 83
alpha-adrenoceptor blockers 128
5-alpha-reductase enzyme 163
amenorrhea
  hypothalamic 156
  primary 156, 158–60
  secondary 156–7
amiloride 123
aminoglutethimide 106, 143
amiodarone 12, 20, 26, *26*
  thyroid dysfunction 26, *26*
androgen insensitivity 158, 167
androgens
  adrenal 104, 136, 137–8, 140
  suppression 139
  biosynthesis 114, 136, 137
  ovarian 150
  replacement 119, 164
'andropause' 163
androstenedione 150
angiotensin receptor blockers 44

angiotensin-converting enzyme (ACE)
inhibitors 44, 47
antiandrogens 152
antidiuretic hormone (ADH/vasopressin)
111–12, *111*
apolipoproteins 171, *171*
apoplexy, pituitary 110
arcus juvenilis *175, 177*
arthritis, degenerative in acromegaly 103
Asherman's syndrome 156
atenolol 128
atherosclerosis 170, 172–3, 178–9
in diabetes mellitus 57–8
role of lipoprotein (a) 187
athersclerotic plaques 58, 172–3
rupture 58
atorvostatin *185*
atrial fibrillation 14
auricular calcification 108
autoantibodies
adrenal 118
pituitary 108
thyroid 15, 22
autoimmune adrenalitis 115
autoimmune disease, thyroid 14–19, 22–4,
204
autoimmune oophoritis 161
autoimmune polyglandular syndromes 75,
115, 204–5
autoimmune regulator gene (AIRE) 204
autonomic neuropathy, diabetes 45, 46, 47

B-cell lymphoma, thyroid 35
basal ganglia, calcification 76
beta-blockers 14, 24, 47, 128
[131]I-6 beta-iodomethyl-norcholesterol
([131]I-NP-59) 144
bilateral macronodular adrenal hyperplasia
(BMAH) 130, 134–5
bile acid sequestrants *185*, 186
bisphosphonates
hyperparathyroidism 74
osteoporosis 70
Paget's disease 82
side-effects 82
bladder, neurogenic 46
blood pressure
aldosteronism 121, 123
control in diabetes 42, 44

pheochromocytoma 125
BMD, *see* bone mineral density
body weight, low 156
bone biopsies
Paget's disease 78–9
rickets 84
sclerotic bone 89
bone densitometry 68, 77
bone marrow failure 87
bone marrow transplantation 89
bone metastases 87
bone mineral density (BMD)
normal 66
osteoporosis 66, 70
brachydactyly 76
breast cancer
bone metastases 87
male 167
breast tissue, male 166
bromocriptine 97, 107, 155
in pregnancy 98
buffalo hump 134
bullae, diabetic 53

C-cells 10, 11
hyperplasia (CCH) 198, 199
cabergoline 97, 155
CAH, *see* congenital adrenal hyperplasia
calcitonin
endogenous 10
MTC 198
osteoporosis 70
Paget's disease 82
side-effects 82
calcitriol (1, 25-dihydroxyvitamin D) 71,
77, 83, 86
calcium
decreased serum 77
intake 69
intravenous therapy 77
raised serum 72
urinary 77
calcium channel blockers 128
calcium sensing receptor agonists
(calcimimmetic agents) 74
candidiasis 51
mucocutaneous 204, 205
carbimazole 14
carcinoid syndrome 202–3

carcinoid tumors 106, 191
cardiac disorders
    carcinoid 202
    dopamine agonists 98
    hyperthyroidism 14
    *see also* cardiovascular disease
cardiovascular disease
    diabetes mellitus 46, 47, 57–9
    lipid disorders 170, 182–4
    reduction with therapy 184
    prevention post-menopause 161
    risk assessment 183–4
Carney complex 28, 132
carotenoderma 20
carotid artery disease 57
catecholamines, excess 125–6
Charcot foot 54–5
chemosis 16
chemotherapy, adrenocortical carcinoma
    143
chlorpropamide 112
cholecalciferol 71, 86
cholesterol absorption inhibitors *185*, 186
cholesterol emboli syndrome 179–80
cholesterol ester transfer protein (CETP),
    inhibition 187
cholesterol, total
    definitions for elevated 170
    therapy for lowering 82–7
cholestyramine *185*, 186
chromogranin A 192, 203
Chvostek's sign 77
chylomicronemia syndrome *174–5*
chylomicrons 171
claudication 56
clitoromegaly 141
clonidine suppression test 126
colesevelam *185*, 186
colestipol *185*, 186
colon polyps 102
computed tomography (CT)
    adrenal incidentaloma 144
    adrenocortical carcinoma 140, 141
    pheochromocytoma 127
    thyroid 29, 37
congenital adrenal hyperplasia (CAH)
    136–9
cornea
    calcium deposits (band keratopathy) 72

lipid deposits 177, 178
corticosteroid-binding globulin (CBG) 119
corticosteroids
    adrenal insufficiency 119
    aldosteronism 123
    CAH 139
    Reidel's thyroiditis 25
cortisol
    24-hour urinary 104, 146
    biosynthesis 136
    reduced 137
    serum 119
    adrenal incidentaloma 146
    morning concentrations 118
cortisol-releasing hormone (CRH),
    stimulation test 104
cosyntropin (ACTH) stimulation test 117,
    118, 139
cotton wool spots 41
Cowden's syndrome 28
cranial mononeuropathies, diabetes 47
craniopharyngioma 111, 112
creatinine, serum 44
critically ill patient, adrenal insufficiency
    119
cryptorchidism 164
Cushing syndrome
    adrenal 130–5, 140, 146
    clinical presentation 132–5
    diabetes mellitus 62–3
    differential diagnosis 135
    management 137
    pituitary 62, 104–6, 130, 131
    subclinical 134, 146
cyclin D1 gene 71
CYP11B1 gene 120, 139
CYP11B2 gene 120
CYP17 gene 139
CYP21A2 gene 139
cytochrome P450 enzymes 137
cytochrome P450 gene mutations 137, 139

Dalrymple sign 16
dehydroepiandrosterone (DHEA) 114,
    119
dehydroepiandrosterone sulfate (DHEAS)
    114, 135, 138–9, 150
dental hypoplasia 76, 84

dermopathy
  diabetic 50
  thyroid-associated 16
desmopressin (DDAVP) 111, 112
dexamethasone 123, 139
dexamethasone suppression test 104, 106, 146
diabetes insipidus, central 111–12
diabetes mellitus
  in acromegaly 60–1
  blood pressure control 42
  cardiovascular disease 46, 47, 57–9
  foot problems 54–6
  nephropathy 43–4
  neuropathy 45–7
  retinopathy 41–2
  skin manifestations 48–53
  type 1 40, 48, 204
  type 2 40, 41, 152
  therapeutic options 59, 64
diarrhea, carcinoid syndrome 202, 203
diet, modification in lipid disorders 184
DiGeorge syndrome 75
1,25-dihydroxy vitamin D (calcitriol) 71, 77, 83, 86
diiodotyrosine (DIT) 10
distal sensorimotor polyneuropathy (DPN) 45
dopamine 92
dopamine agonists 97–8, 107, 155
  prolactinoma 97–8
  side-effects 98
doxazosin 128
drug eruptions, diabetic therapies 52
drugs
  affecting thyroid hormone binding *11*
  avoidance before metanephrine/catecholamine measurement *126*
  causing gynecomastia *166*
  causing hyperprolactinemia 154
  causing hypothyroidism 20
  causing osteoporosis *67*
  causing thyroiditis 26
  iodine-containing 12
dual energy X-ray absorptiometry 68, 69
dysbetalipoproteinemia *174–5*, 179

edema, periorbital 16
elderly, hypothyroidism 21
empty sell syndrome 109
empty sella syndrome 108, 109
endometriosis 152, 153
endothelin-1 87
enzyme deficiencies
  CAH 136
  hypogonadism 163
eplerenone 122, 123
erectile dysfunction, diabetic neuropathy 47
ergocalciferol 74, 86
erythema, necrolytic migratory 63–4
esophageal motility disorders 46
estrogen 161
  in male 166
estrogen replacement 160, 161
  hyperparathyroidism 74
  osteoporosis 70
etomidate 143
eunochoid body habitus 164, 165
exercise
  intensive 156
  and osteoporosis 69
exophthalmos 16, 17, 18
eye disease
  diabetic 41–2
  hyperparathyroidism 72
  lipid disorders 177, 178, 179
  thyroid disease 12, 16, 17
ezetimibe *185*, 186

facial features
  acromegaly 60, 61, 100
  Addison's disease 116
  Cushing syndrome 63, 133, 134
  GH-secreting adenoma 95
  MEN2B 197
fallopian tube disorders 152–3
familial combined hyperlipidemia (FCH) *174–5*
familial defective apoB-100 (FDB) *174–5*
familial hyperaldosteronism type I 120
familial hypercholesterolemia *174–5*
familial hypoalphalipoproteinemia *176–7*
familial hypobetalipoproteinemia *176–7*
familial medullary thyroid cancer (FMTC) 196, 199

feet
  in diabetes 47
  in lipid disorders 180
feminization, males 140
fenofibrate *185*
fibric acids *185*, 186
fibroids 153
fine-needle aspiration (FNA)
  adrenal incidentaloma 145
  thyroid 25, 36–7, 198
  thyroid nodule 28–9
fish oils *185*, 186
flame hemorrhages 41
fludrocortisone 119, 139
fluorescein angiography 42
flushing 202
flutamide 152
fluvastatin *185*
foam cells 57, 172
folic acid 187
follicle stimulating hormone (FSH) *93*
  elevation 156, 161
  female infertility 152
  hypogonadism 164
foot
  in acromegaly 101
  diabetic 54–6
fractures
  greenstick 86
  osteopetrosis 88
  osteoporotic 66
fragile X syndrome 156, 161
Framingham scoring 183–4
funduscopy
  diabetic retinopathy 41–2
  lipid disorders 179, 180

G-protein coupled receptors 132
galactorrhea 154, 155
gamma knife 103
Gardner's syndrome 28
gastrinoma 190, 192
gastrointestinal diseases
  adrenal insufficiency 117, *117*
  causing osteoporosis *67*
  diabetes 46, 47
gemifibrozil *185*
genitalia, ambiguous 138, 139
gingival mucosa, hyperpigmentation 116

glitazone 59
glomerular basement membrane (GBM) 43
glucagonoma 63–4, 192–4
glucocorticoid-remediable aldosteronism
    (GRA) 120, 121
glucocorticoids 123, 139
  deficiency 115–19
  replacement 119
glucorticoid antagonists 106
glucose tolerance test, oral 102
glyburide 59
goiter
  Graves' disease 16
  thyroiditis 22
gonadal dysgenesis, primary 158, 160
gonadotrophin-releasing hormone
    (GnRH) 163
gonadotrophins
  deficiency 109
  *see also named gonadotrophins*
Graves' disease 12, 13, 14–19, 28
greenstick fractures 86
growth factors, diabetic nephropathy 43
growth hormone (GH) *93*, 95
  deficiency 109
growth hormone (GH)-secreting tumors
    60–1, 95
growth-hormone-releasing hormone
    (GHRH) 60
gynecomastia 165, 166–7

hands
  in acromegaly 101
  hypoparathyroidism 76
  rickets 85
  skin hyperpigmentation 116
  thyroid acropachy 16, 18
  xanthomas 176, 179, 181
Hashimoto's thyroiditis 22–3
headaches *93*, 107, 110, 121, 125
high density lipoproteins (HDLs) 171, 173
  definitions for elevated *170*
  therapy for raising 187
Hirschsprung's disease 196
hirsutism 138, 150, 151, 152
homocysteine 187
'hook effect' phenomenon 97
hormone receptors, Cushing syndrome
    etiology 132

hormone replacement therapy
  osteoporosis 70
  primary hyperparathyroidism 74
hormone-releasing hormones 92
Hurthle cell thyroid cancer 34
hydrocortisone 119, 139
18-hydroxycorticosterone 122
5-hydroxyindoleacetic acid (5-HIAA) 203
21-hydroxylase deficiency 136, 137, 138–9
11β-hydroxylase deficiency 136, 139
17α-hydroxylase deficiency 136, 139
17α-hydroxyprogesterone (17-OHP) 137,
  138–9
5-hydroxytryptophan (5-HTP) 203
hymen, imperforate 158, 159
hyperaldosteronism 120–3
  familial type I 120
  idiopathic (IHA) 120, 122
hypercalcemia 72
hypercholesterolemia
  definitions 170
  etiology 170
  familial 170, *174–5*
  therapies 182–7
hyperglycemia
  and cardiovascular disease 57, 58
  nephropathy 43
  neuropathy 45
  retinopathy 41
hyperlipoproteinemia, type III *174–5*
hypernatremia 121
hyperostosis frontalis interna 76
hyperparathyroidism
  in MEN1 190, 192
  in MEN2 201
  primary 71–4
  secondary 71, 74
hyperpigmentation 106, 116, *117*
hyperprolactinemia 96, 97, 154–5
  clinical presentation 96, *96*, 154
  differential diagnosis *97*, 154
  hypogonadism 154, 163, 164
  iatrogenic 154
  idiopathic 154
  management 155
  pituitary tumors 154
hypersensitivity reactions, insulin
  preparations 52

hypertension
  Cushing syndrome 134
  diabetes 42, 44
  pheochromocytoma 125
  primary aldosteronism 121, 123
hyperthyroidism 12–14
  subclinical 14
hypobetalipoproteinemia, familial *176–7*
hypocalcemia, causing secondary
  hyperparathyroidism 71, 74
hypogonadism 154, 163–5
  congenital secondary 163
  hyperprolactinemia 154, 163, 164
  hypopituitarism 109
  hypothalamic 162, 163
  time of onset 164
hypokalemia 120, 121, 122, 134
hypolipoproteinemias *176–7*
hypoparathyroidism 25, 75–7
hypophosphatasia 83
hypophosphatemia, rickets 83, 86
hypopituitarism 107–8, 109, 110
  acute decompensation 110
hypothalamic amenorrhea 156
hypothalamic hormones *93*
hypothalamic–pituitary–ovarian (HPO) axis
  152
hypothalamic–pituitary–thyroid axis 10
hypothalamus 92
hypothyroidism 20–1
  subclinical 21

ileal bypass, partial 186
immunosuppressive therapy 205
infections
  causing adrenal insufficiency 115, *115*
  causing testicular failure 163
  diabetes mellitus 50, 51
inferior petrosal sinus sampling 106
infertility
  female 152–3
  male 162
inhibin 161, 163
insulin resistance 40
  in PCOS 150, 152
insulin sensitizers 52, 59, 150
insulin therapy 59
  pumps 52
  reactions 52

insulin tolerance test (ITT) 118
insulin-like growth factor-1 (IGF-1) 41,
     60, 102
   binding protein-3 60
insulin-like growth factor-2 (IGF-2) 140
insulinoma 192, 193
interferon 20, 26, 64
interleukin-2 (IL-2) 26
intertrigo 51
iodine
   deficiency 20
   excess 12, 20, *26*
   *see also* radioactive iodine
islet cell tumors 63, 106, 191, 194, 195

Jansen's chondrodystrophy 75
Jod–Basedow disease 12
joint mobility, diabetes mellitus 54

Kallman's syndrome 158, 163
karyotype
   male hypogonadism 165
   Turner's syndrome 158, 160
keratopathy, band 72
ketoconazole 106, 135, 143
Klinfelter's syndrome 163, 164, 165
kyphosis 69

lanreotide 61, 64
Laurence–Moon–Biedel syndrome 163
levothyroxine (LT4) 21, 22
Leydig cells 163
lid retraction, thyroid disease 16, 17
Liddle's sign 134
lifestyle modification 184
lipemia retinalis *175, 178, 179*
lipid disorders
   clinical presentation 173–80
   definitions 170, *170*
   diagnosis 182
   differential diagnosis 181–2
   etiology and pathophysiology 170–3
   hyperlipoproteinemias *174–5*
   hypolipoproteinemias *176–7*
   management 182–7
lipoatrophy 52
lipohypertrophy 52
lipoprotein (a) 187
lithium 20, 26, *67*

livedo reticularis 180
liver
   carcinoids 203
   lipid metabolism 172–3
   MTC metastases 200
liver failure 166
long bones
   Paget's disease 80, 81
   rickets 84–6
lovastatin *185*
low density lipoprotein (LDL) cholesterol
     57, *170*
   definition of elevated *170*
   goals and cutpoints for therapy *183*
   reduction therapies 182–6
LT4, *see* levothyroxine
lung carcinoma, small-cell 62, 105
luteinizing hormone (LH) *93*
luteinizing hormone-releasing hormone
     (LHRH) 92
lymphadenopathy, thyroid disease 18, 37–8
lymphocytic hypophysitis 107–8
lymphoma, thyroid 35

McCune–Albright syndrome 130
macrophages, foam cells 57, 172
macular edema 42
magnetic resonance imaging (MRI)
   adrenal incidentaloma 145
   adrenocortical carcinoma 140, 141
   pheochromocytoma 128
   posterior pituitary 112
   thyroid 29, 37
marfanoid body habitus 197
medullary thyroid carcinoma (MTC) 34
   familial 196, 199
   in MEN2 198–200
β-melanocyte stimulating hormone (β-
     MSH) 106
MEN, *see*, multiple endocrine neoplasia
MEN type 1 gene 71, 190
menarche, absence 158–60
menopause 161
metabolic acidosis 120
$^{123}$I-metaiodobenzylguanidine (MIBG)
     scan 128, 129
metanephrines, plasma 125–6
metaphyses, widening 85, 86

metformin
   diabetes 52, 59
   PCOS 152
methimazole 14
methotrexate 25
metyrapone 106, 135, 143
microalbuminuria 43
microaneurisms 41
microphallus 164, 165
mifepristone 106
mineralocorticoids 139
   deficiency 115–19
   replacement 119
mitotane 106, 135, 143
moniodotyrosine (MIT) 10
mortality, acromegaly 102
mucormycosis 50
mullerian-inhibiting hormone 158
multiple endocrine neoplasia type 1 (MEN 1)
   64, 71, 190–5
   clinical presentation 190–1
   etiology and pathophysiology 190, 191
   management 192–5
   tumor expression testing 194, *195*
multiple endocrine neoplasia type 2A/2B
   (MEN2A/2B) 34, 71, 196–201
   medullary thyroid cancer 198–200
   pheochromocytoma 124–5, 200–1
   primary hyperparathyroidism 201
muscular dystrophy 163
myelolipoma 144, 145
myocardial infarction (MI) 57, 58, 179
myopathy, Cushing syndrome 134
myxedema 20
   pretibial 16, 17
myxedema coma 20, 21

necrobiosis lipoidica diabeticorum 48
nephrolithiasis 72, 73, 201
nephropathy, diabetic 43–4
neurofibromatosis type 1 (NF-1) 124
neuromas, in MEN2B 196, 197
neuropathy, diabetic 45–7
niacin 187
nicotinic acids *185*, 186
nuclear factor-κβ (NF-κβ) pathway 78

obesity 166
octreotide 61, 64, 102, 106, 107, 203

octreotide scanning 128, 203
omega-3-fatty acids *185*, 186
oophoritis, autoimmune 161
ophthalmopathy
   diabetic 41–2, 47
   thyroid-associated 12, 16, 17
ophthalmoplegia 16, 17, 47
optic chiasm 92, 95
osteitis fibrosis 73
osteoblastic bone metastases 87–9
osteoclasts 66, 67
   bone resorption 87
   giant multinucleate 78, 79
osteoid, excess 84
osteomalacia 82–6
osteomyelitis, diabetic foot disease 56
osteopetroses 87
osteoporosis 66–70
osteosarcoma 79
otitis externa, malignant 50
ovaries
   menopausal changes 161
   polycystic syndrome 150–2
   premature failure 152–3, 156, 161
   steroidogenesis 150

PAC:PRA ratio, *see* plasma aldosterone
   concentration/plasma renin activity ratio
Paget's disease 78–82
pain management, diabetic neuropathy 47
pamidronate 82
pancreatic islet cell tumors 63, 106, 191,
   194, 195
parathyroid glands
   adenoma 29, 71–4
   cyst 29
   imaging 72, 73, 74
   multiple in MEN 1 190, 191
parathyroid hormone (PTH)
   human recombinant 70, 77
   low levels 25, 75–7
   raised 71–4, 190, 192
   resistance 75
parathyroidectomy 192
PCOS, *see* polycystic ovary syndrome
pegnisomant 102
pelvic inflammatory disease 152
Pemberton's sign 28, 29
peptic ulcers 190

pergolide mesylate 97, 98
peripheral vascular disease, diabetes 54–6,
  57–9
pheochromocytoma 124–9, 196
  clinical features 125
  diagnosis 125–8
  differential diagnosis 128
  etiology 124–5
  extra-adrenal (paragangliomas) 124
  familial and MEN2A/2B 124–5, 200–1
  malignant 129
  management 128–9
photoallergic reactions 52
photocoagulation 42
pituitary adenoma 92, 93
  ACTH-secreting 104–6, 156
  clinical manifestations *93*
  Cushing disease 62, 130, 131
  GH-secreting 99–103
  hypopituitarism 109
  macroadenoma 94
  MEN1 191, 192, 193
  microadenoma 94, 95
  nonfunctioning/glycoprotein-secreting
  107
  *see also* prolactinoma
pituitary apoplexy 110
pituitary carcinoma 92
pituitary gland
  anatomy 92
  hemorrhagic infarction 110, 156
  lymphocytic hypophysitis 107–8
  posterior 111–12
  trans-sphenoidal resection 61, 98, 106
pituitary hormones 92, *93*
  releasing-hormones 92
*Pityrosporum orbiculare* 51
plasma, lipemic *175*, 178
plasma aldosterone concentration/plasma
  renin activity (PAC:PRA) ratio 122, 146
polycystic ovary syndrome (PCOS) 150–2
polyuria/polydipsia *111*
positron emission tomography (PET) 128,
  144
postpartum pituitary infarction 110
postpartum thyroiditis 22, *23*, 24
posture test 122, 123
PPNAD, *see* primary pigmented nodular
  adrenocortical disease

Prader–Willi syndrome 163
pravastatin *185*
prednisone 123, 139
pregnancy
  bromocriptine therapy 98
  CAH 139
  Graves' disease 19
  hypothyroidism 21
  postpartum Sheehan's syndrome 110
  postpartum thyroiditis 22, *23*, 24
premature ovarian failure (POF) 152–3,
  156, 161
primary pigmented nodular adrenocortical
  disease (PPNAD) 132, 135
progesterone replacement 70, 74
prognathism 95
prolactin (PRL) 92, *93*, 108
  raised serum levels 97, 154–5
  suppression 97–8
prolactinoma 95, 96–8, 154–5
  MEN1 191
propranolol 14, 128
proptosis 16, 17
propylthiouracil 14, 19
prostate cancer 164
  bone metastases 87, 89
prostate specific antigen (PSA) 87
protein kinase C (PKC) 45
proteinuria 43, 44
pseudo-Cushing's state 135
pseudofracture 86, 88
pseudohypoparathyroidism 75–7
*Pseudomonas aeruginosa* 50
pseudovitamin D deficiency 83
pubarche, precocious 150
puberty, gynecomastia 166, 167

radiation therapy
  adrenocortical carcinoma 143
  pituitary macroadenoma 102–3
radioactive iodine scanning
  thyroid cancer 37
  thyroid nodule 28, 29
  thyroiditis 22, 24
  thyrotoxicosis 12, 13
radioactive iodine therapy 19, 38
radiosurgery (gamma knife) 103
raloxifene 70
Reidel's thyroiditis *23*, 25

renal disease
  chronic 71
  in diabetes 43–4
  secondary hyperparathyroidism 71, 74
renal stones 201
renin, plasma activity (PRA) 122, 139
RET proto-oncogene 34, 38, 71, 124–5,
  196
  structure 197
  testing 196
retinopathy, diabetic 41–2
rickets 82–6
Riedel's thyroiditis 23, 25
rosuvastatin *185*

salt loading, oral 122
salt-wasting disease 137, 139
sandostatin 102
scavenger receptor B-1 (SRB-1) 187
Schmidt's syndrome 204
scintigraphy
  adrenal mass 144
  parathyroid glands 72, 73, 74, 192
  *see also* radioactive iodine scanning
sclerotic bone disorders 87–9
sella turica 92
  empty 108, 109
sequestrosome 1 protein 78
serotonin, carcinoid syndrome 202
sestamibi scanning, parathyroid glands 72,
  73, 74, 192
sex-hormone binding globulin (SHBG)
  166
Sheehan's syndrome 110, 156
simvastatin *185*
sinuses, enlargement in acromegaly 100
sitosterolemia *176–7*
skin disorders
  adrenal insufficiency 116
  Cushing syndrome 105, 106, 132, 134
  diabetes mellitus 48–53
  glucagonoma 63–4
  lipid disorders 176, 177, 178
  thyroid disease 16, 17
skin flushing 202
skull, Paget's disease 79, 80
somatostatin analogs 61, 64, 102, 203
somatostatin receptor imaging 128
sperm abnormalities 162

spine
  osteoporosis 69
  Paget's disease 80
  vertebral overgrowth 103
spironolactone 122, 123, 152
  side-effects 123
statins 184, *185*
steroidogenic acute regulatory protein
  (StAR) deficiency 136
steroids, biosynthesis 136, 150
Stevens–Johnson syndrome 52
'streak gonad' 158
streptozotosin 143
striae, Cushing syndrome 104, 105, 132,
  134
sulfonylureas 52, 59

T-cell lymphoma, thyroid 35
T3, *see* triiodothyronine
T4, *see* thyroxine
tamoxifen 25, 167
Tangier disease *176–7*, 181–2
tartrate resistant acid phosphatase (TRAP)
  87
teeth, enamel hypoplasia 76, 84
telangiectasias 48
tendons, xanthomas *175*, 176, 181
teriparatide 70
testicular adrenal rests 138
testicular function, regulation 163
testosterone 163
  biosynthesis 136, 137
  disorders of action 163
  ovarian 150
  replacement therapy 164
thiazides 112
thiazolidendiones 52, 152
thionamides 14, 19
thirst *111*
thymectomy 192
thyroglobulin (Tg) 10, 22, 38
  antibodies 22
thyroid cancer 30, 31
  anaplastic 35, 38
  clinical presentation 35–6
  diagnosis 36–7
  follicular cell 34
  Hurthle cell 34
  lymphoma 35

management 37–8
medullary 34, 198–200
papillary 31–3
thyroid gland
anatomy 10
autoimmune disease 14–19, 22–4, 204
FNA 25, 28–9, 36–7, 198
histology
Graves' disease 15
nodules 28–9
normal 10, 11
thyroiditis 23, 24, 25
thyroid hormones 10, *11*
replacement 21
thyroiditis 22–3
thyroid microsomal peroxidase (TPO) 10
antibodies 22, 24, 26
thyroid nodules 26–30
clinical presentation 26–8
investigations 28–9
treatment 30
thyroid-stimulating hormone (TSH) 10
deficiency 109
hypothyroidism 20, 21
levels after radioiodine ablation 38
receptor autoantibodies (TSHRAbs) 15, 19
subclinical hyperthyroidism 14
thyrotoxicosis 12
thyroid-stimulating hormone (TSH)-
secreting adenoma 107
thyroidectomy 30
Graves' disease 19
MTC 200
subtotal 19
in thyroid cancer 37
thyroiditis 14, 22
drug-induced 26, *26*
Hashimoto's 22–3
painful subacute *23*, 24, 25
painless 24
postpartum 22, *23*, 24
Reidel's *23*, 25
suppurative *23*, 24
syndromes *22, 23*
thyrotoxicosis 12–14
'apathetic' 12
thyroiditis 22, 24

thyroxine (T4)
free T4 levels 14, 18, 20
synthesis 10
T4 index 20
tinea infections 51
tongue, hyperpigmentation 116
tonsils, Tangier disease 181–2
trachea, deviation/compression in thyroid disease 26–8
transforming growth factor-β (TGF-β) 25, 43, 45
triglycerides 171
definitions for elevated *170*
triiodothyronine (T3) 10
intravenous 21
Trosseau's sign 77
tuberculosis 118
Turner's syndrome 156, 157, 158–60

ulcers, diabetic foot 54–6
ultrasound, thyroid gland 28
urine
aldosterone excretion 122, 146
calcium 77
cortisol 104, 146
osmolality 112
uterus, diseases and anomalies 152–3, 158, 160

'vanishing testes syndrome' 158
varicocele 162
vascular endothelial growth factor (VEGF) 42, 43, 45
vasopressin (antidiuretic hormone/ADH) 111–12, *111*
VEGF, *see* vascular endothelial growth factor
venous congestion, thyroid nodules 26–8
venous thrombosis, glucagonoma 64
vertebrae, overgrowth in acromegaly 103
very low density lipoproteins (VLDLs) 171, 172
virilization
female 134, 135, 137–8, 140, 150, 151
inadequate male 163, 164–5
virus particles, Paget's disease etiology 78
visual field defects 95, *96*, 107, 110
vitamin $B_6$ 187

vitamin D 69
    congenital errors of metabolism 83
    deficiency 71, 74, 83
vitiligo 116, *117*, 157
von Basedow's disease, *see* Graves' disease
von Hippel–Lindau (VHL) disease 124

water deprivation test 112
weight loss *117*
Wolff–Chiakoff effect 20
Womens' Health Initiative study 161

X-linked hypophosphatemic rickets 83
xanthelasmas *175*, 177
xanthoma
    cutaneous 176
    eruptive *175*, 178
    palmar *175*, 179
    tendon *175*, 176, 181
    tuberous *175*

zoledronic acid 82, 89
zygomycosis 50